Psychic Retreats

Essentially clinical in its approach, *Psychic Retreats* discusses the problem of patients who are stuck and with whom it is difficult to make meaningful contact. John Steiner, an experienced psychiatrist and psychoanalyst, uses new developments in Kleinian theory to explain how this happens. He examines the way object relationships and defences can be organized into complex structures which lead to a personality and an analysis becoming rigid and stuck, with little opportunity for development or change. These systems of defences are pathological organizations of the personality: John Steiner describes them as 'psychic retreats', into which the patient can withdraw to avoid contact both with the analyst and with reality.

To provide a background to these original and controversial concepts, the author builds on more established ideas, such as Klein's distinction between the paranoid–schizoid and depressive positions, and briefly reviews previous work on pathological organizations of the personality. He illustrates his discussion with detailed clinical material, including examples of the way psychic retreats operate to provide a respite from both paranoid–schizoid and depressive anxieties. He looks at the way such organizations function as a defence against unbearable guilt and describes the mechanism by which fragmentation of the personality can be reversed so that lost parts of the self can be regained and reintegrated into the personality.

Psychic Retreats is written with practising psychoanalysts and psycho-analytic psychotherapists in mind; the emphasis is therefore clinical throughout the book, which concludes with a chapter on the technical problems which arise in the treatment of such severely ill patients.

John Steiner is a member of the British Psycho–Analytical Society and a Consultant Psychotherapist at the Tavistock Clinic, London.

THE NEW LIBRARY OF PSYCHOANALYSIS

The New Library of Psychoanalysis was launched in 1987 in association with the Institute of Psycho-Analysis, London. Its purpose is to facilitate a greater and more widespread appreciation of what psychoanalysis is really about and to provide a forum for increasing mutual understanding between psychoanalysts and those working in other disciplines such as history, linguistics, literature, medicine, philosophy, psychology, and the social sciences. It is intended that the titles selected for publication in the series should deepen and develop psychoanalytic thinking and technique, contribute to psychoanalysis from outside or contribute to other disciplines from a psychoanalytical perspective.

The Institute, together with the British Psycho-Analytical Society, runs a low-fee psychoanalytic clinic, organizes lectures and scientific events concerned with psychoanalysis, publishes the *International Journal of Psycho-Analysis*, and runs the only training course in the UK in psychoanalysis leading to membership of the International Psychoanalytical Association – the body which preserves internationally agreed standards of training, of professional entry, and of professional ethics and practice for psychoanalysis as initiated and developed by Sigmund Freud. Distinguished members of the Institute have included Michael Balint, Wilfred Bion, Ronald Fairbairn, Anna Freud, Ernest Jones, Melanie Klein, John Rickman, and Donald Winnicott.

Volumes 1–11 in the series have been prepared under the general editorship of David Tuckett, with Ronald Britton and Eglé Laufer as associate editors. Subsequent volumes are under the general editorship of Elizabeth Bott Spillius, with, from Volume 17, Donald Campbell, Michael Parsons, Rosine Jozef Perelberg and David Taylor as associate editors.

ALSO IN THIS SERIES

NEW LIBRARY OF PSYCHOANALYSIS
—— 19 ——

General editor: Elizabeth Bott Spillius

Psychic Retreats

Pathological Organizations in Psychotic, Neurotic and Borderline Patients

JOHN STEINER

Foreword by Roy Schafer

First published 1993
by Routledge
11 New Fetter Lane, London EC4P 4EE

Simultaneously published in the USA and Canada
by Routledge
29 West 35th Street, New York, NY 10001

Routledge is an imprint of the Taylor & Francis group

Reprinted 1994, 1995, 1998 and 1999

© 1993 John Steiner

Typeset in Bembo by LaserScript, Mitcham, Surrey
Printed and bound in Great Britain by
Mackays of Chatham PLC, Chatham Kent

British Library Cataloguing in Publication Data
A catalogue record for this book is available from the British Library

Library of Congress Cataloging in Publication Data
A catalogue record for this book is available from the British Library

ISBN 0–415–09923–4 (hbk)
ISBN 0–415–09924–2 (pbk)

Contents

Acknowledgements

I would like to offer thanks to my family and to my colleagues at the British Psycho-Analytical Society and the Tavistock Clinic for their help and support. Versions of the manuscript were read and commented on by Michael Feldman, Ronald Britton, Hanna Segal, Priscilla Roth, Betty Joseph and by my wife Deborah Steiner. Their comments were invaluable. Elizabeth Spillius played a vital role as an editor, colleague and friend. Special gratitude is owed to my patients, both those whose material appears in this book and the others who helped in the development and clarification of my ideas.

Foreword

ROY SCHAFER

One can only admire the fine empathy, subtle understanding, impressive patience and refreshing candour that run through these pages. Beyond admiration, however, any careful reading of John Steiner's work should add significantly to the clinical resourcefulness of analyst and psychotherapist alike. Of particular value is Steiner's interpretive approach to the inevitably painful and disheartening stretches in therapeutic work with deeply disturbed patients – just the kind of work that, throughout our careers, we mental health professionals must confront time and time again.

Steiner convincingly portrays a subgroup of these difficult-to-treat patients as unable to tolerate the pain of either the paranoid-schizoid position or the depressive position. Consequently, they take refuge from the world of real relationships; they establish for themselves psychic retreats within which they feel protected even though often still in pain. In a perverse way, they even seem to be able to find narcissistic and masochistic gratifications in these retreats. This they do by erecting pathological organizations of defences and fantasized object relations, using for their building materials a goodly amount of projective identification, idealization, serious compromise of their sense of reality and, for the sake of a sense of safety, abject submission to the very organization that they have contrived in the internal world. Understandably, then, they experience the therapist's interventions as both threatening their safety and limiting their gratifications, and so they set themselves against the very person to whom they have turned for help.

In large part these patients have retreated from the painful difficulties that lie in the way of their mourning the loss that must be experienced when they separate from their primitively conceived internal objects. Steiner has much to teach about the experiences of devastation that often accompany mourning the 'loss' of objects from whom, psychically, one is separating. Equally instructive in his delineation of the counter-transferences that are certain to be stimulated as the analyst or therapist feels enticed into this strange, ambivalent alternative world of unconscious phantasy; then, various kinds of insensitivity and collusion are virtually unavoidable. These counter-transferences can be put to good use as they come to be understood and mastered.

Steiner shows all this in both his commentary on a number of vivid, detailed clinical examples and his brilliant concluding essay on the effects of different ways of framing interpretations. How we address these patients, particularly in times of painful impasse, can make a big difference in our effectiveness. These clinical examples and reflections exemplify some of the finest analytic work being done today. They should help us to think our way through difficult periods in our work with every sort of patient, not just those in the subgroup singled out by the author.

Steiner brings to bear ideas drawn from a broad knowledge of the psychoanalytic literature, in which regard he is appealingly modest in what he claims for himself. His debt to Freud shows everywhere as does his debt to many great pioneers in psychoanalysis, particularly those who have been more or less identified with, and major contributors to, Kleinian thinking, among them Herbert Rosenfeld, Wilfred Bion, Hanna Segal and Betty Joseph. But his scholarship is broader than just this much, which is all to the good for those readers who are not committed Kleinian therapists or analysts; for on this basis they should find many points of entry into the clinical examples and discussions.

Because so many of us in the field of mental healing find ourselves up against the pathological organizations that John Steiner has devoted himself to identifying and understanding psychoanalytically, *Psychic Retreats* will surely soon establish itself as a necessary addition to every clinician's bookshelf. To use the phrase that he turns to such good advantage in his absorbing essay on the Oedipus plays of Sophocles, none of us can afford to 'turn a blind eye' to work of this high quality.

Introduction

The themes discussed in this book developed out of my struggle to think about practical difficulties in the analysis of several patients. In common with many contemporary analysts two problems occupied me in particular, first that of making meaningful contact with my patients and second that of coping with analyses which became repetitive, static and unproductive. Experiences with such patients led to the observation that they used a variety of mechanisms to create states of mind which provided protection from anxiety and pain. They retreated out of contact with the analyst into these states which were often experienced spatially as if they were places in which the patient could hide. I have come to refer to them as psychic retreats, refuges, shelters, sanctuaries or havens and this book is about the way they operate. If such states of withdrawal are prolonged and repetitive development is seriously impeded and the analysis tends to become stuck. This leads to a clinical situation which raises questions about the analyst's technique, including his or her capacity for understanding, as well as issues of the patient's psychopathology and selection of defences, and these will be considered in the following chapters.

In Chapter 1 I introduce some of the main themes of the book by presenting an outline of a theory of psychic retreats, including the central idea that they reflect the activity of pathological organizations of the personality. These organizations are conceptualized both as a grouping of defences and as a highly structured, close-knit system of object relationships. Although this chapter is rather theoretical my orientation is primarily clinical and my concern is to understand the patient and the analyst as they interact in the analytic consulting room. However, theory is not only important and interesting in its own right but should be clinically useful as well. Since the analyst always has a theory, whether he[1]

---

1 Throughout this book I have tried to avoid sexist language, but I sometimes use 'he' to refer to an analyst or patient of either sex for the sake of simplicity and clarity.

consciously espouses one or not, in my view, it is better to have a conscious theory than an unconscious prejudice. It is important to emphasize, however, that the theoretical descriptions I elaborate are intended to provide a background orientation and are not meant to be applied as formulas in the consulting room when one is actually with the patient. Here I agree with Bion (1970) that the primary task of the analyst is to make himself available for the patient and to open his mind to receive his communications with as little interference as possible. Theory, like 'memory and desire', can fill the analyst's mind and leave insufficient room for the patient's projections. However, a sound theoretical approach making use of simple and clear theories when thinking about clinical material between sessions, in writing and in discussion with colleagues, actually makes it easier for the theory to recede into the background when one is with the patient.

In Chapter 2 I describe psychic retreats in more detail and use clinical material to illustrate the way they operate and act as a refuge from both paranoid–schizoid and depressive anxieties.

Chapter 3 presents a review of the paranoid–schizoid and the depressive positions and the anxieties characteristic of each. These are subdivided further to clarify points at which the individual is under particular stress and, as a result, is likely to turn to the protection of a pathological organization of the personality.

Chapter 4 continues the review to cover narcissistic object relations, and previous work on pathological organizations of the personality. Although this review concentrates on Kleinian authors it is important to recognize that many analysts other than Kleinian ones have done important work in this and related areas sometimes using similar concepts but different terminology. It was not possible to fully review this work but in Chapter 4 some of it is briefly discussed.

Chapter 5 describes the way parts of the self lost through projective identification are recovered. The reversibility of projective identification and the recovery of parts of the self lost through this mechanism are central when moves away from the retreat are considered. The normal sequence of events which constitute mourning is reviewed in this chapter and a model is described which suggests that it is through the process of mourning that parts of the self are regained.

Chapter 6 discusses psychotic organizations. The psychotic patient's need to repair his ego arises from a desperate situation, the aftermath of an internal catastrophe in which his own mind has been attacked. The way pathological organizations of the personality serve as a patch over the damaged ego is explained.

Chapter 7 illustrates the way a pathological organization is brought into play when the patient feels wronged and resentful but cannot give expression to his wish for revenge. The organization may again act as a defence against persecution and fragmentation but at the same time it can come to protect the patient from depressive pain and guilt and prevent the experience of loss. If the patient is able to emerge from the psychic retreat to make contact with psychic reality he may be able to recognize sufficient good feelings to enable him to feel regret and remorse. If this happens, mourning is able to proceed and projections can be withdrawn from the object and returned to the self. The patient feels he is capable of being forgiven and in turn can forgive so that moves towards reparation can be embarked on.

Chapter 8 discusses perverse aspects of psychic retreats and examines the special type of relationship with reality which is characteristic of them. I suggest here that reality is dealt with by being simultaneously accepted and disavowed in the manner which Freud described in his study of fetishism (Freud 1927).

Chapter 9 extends this discussion by illustrating how perverse object relations, including perverse relationships between parts of the self, help to strengthen the hold pathological organizations have on the personality.

In Chapter 10 I turn to literature and look at Sophocles' great plays about Oedipus, which have had such a profound influence on psycho-analysis. I use this material to look at two types of psychic retreat. In *Oedipus the King* I describe perverse mechanisms, particularly what I call 'turning a blind eye', which enables the truth to be both acknowl-edged and disavowed, that is, to be known and not known at the same time. In *Oedipus at Colonus* a more radical rupture with reality has taken place which I refer to as a 'flight from truth to omnipotence' and this serves as an example of a psychotic type of retreat.

Finally in Chapter 11 some of the technical problems presented in analysis by patients in the grip of a pathological organization of the personality are discussed. There I suggest that it is useful to distinguish between the 'need for understanding' and the 'need to be understood'. On this basis it is possible schematically to divide transference inter-pretations into those which are patient-centred and those which are analyst-centred. I discuss the advantages and disadvantages of each and suggest that sometimes, in patients with a powerful propensity to withdraw to psychic retreats, patient-centred interpretations can be particularly intrusive and persecuting. At these times a shift to analyst-centred interpretations may help the analyst to understand what is going on and, sometimes, to avoid an impasse.

1

A theory of psychic retreats

A psychic retreat provides the patient with an area of relative peace and protection from strain when meaningful contact with the analyst is experienced as threatening. It is not difficult to understand the need for transient withdrawal of this kind, but serious technical problems arise in patients who turn to a psychic retreat, habitually, excessively, and indiscriminately. In some analyses, particularly with borderline and psychotic patients, a more or less permanent residence in the retreat may be taken up and it is then that obstacles to development and growth arise.

In my own clinical experience this type of withdrawal and the resultant failure to allow contact with the analyst takes many forms. An aloof type of schizoid superiority is expressed as a cold condescension in one patient and as a mocking dismissal of my work in another. Some patients are clearly reacting to anxiety, and their withdrawal appears to indicate that the analysis has touched on a sensitive topic which has to be avoided. Perhaps the most difficult type of retreat is that in which a false type of contact is offered and the analyst is invited to engage in ways which seem superficial, dishonest, or perverse. Sometimes these reactions can be seen to result from clumsy or intrusive behaviour on the part of the analyst, but it often happens that even careful analysis leaves the patients out of contact. They retreat behind a powerful system of defences which serve as a protective armour or hiding place, and it is sometimes possible to observe how they emerge with great caution like a snail coming out of its shell and retreat once more if contact leads to pain or anxiety.

We have come to understand that obstacles to contact and obstacles to progress and development are related, and that they both arise from the deployment of a particular type of defensive organization by means of which the patient hopes to avoid intolerable anxiety. I call such

1

systems of defences '*pathological organizations of the personality*' and use this term to denote a family of defensive systems which are characterized by extremely unyielding defences and which function to help the patient to avoid anxiety by avoiding contact with other people and with reality. The pursuit of this approach has led me to examine in more detail the way defences operate and, in particular, how they interconnect to form complex, closely knit defensive systems.

The analyst observes psychic retreats as states of mind in which the patient is stuck, cut off, and out of reach, and he may infer that these states arise from the operation of a powerful system of defences. The patient's view of the retreat is reflected in the descriptions which he gives and also in unconscious phantasy as it is revealed in dreams, memories, and reports from everyday life which give a pictorial or dramatized image of how the retreat is unconsciously experienced. Typically it appears as a house, a cave, a fortress, a desert island, or a similar location which is seen as an area of relative safety. Alternatively, it can take an inter-personal form, usually as an organization of objects or part-objects which offers to provide security. It may be represented as a business organization, as a boarding school, as a religious sect, as a totalitarian government or a Mafia-like gang. Often tyrannical and perverse elements are evident in the description, but sometimes the organization is idealized and admired.

Usually over a period of time various representations can be observed which help to build up a picture of the patient's defensive organization. Later I will try to show that it is sometimes useful to think of it as a grouping of object relations, defences, and phantasies which makes up a borderline position similar to but distinct from the paranoid–schizoid and the depressive positions described by Melanie Klein (1952).

The relief provided by the retreat is achieved at the cost of isolation, stagnation, and withdrawal, and some patients find such a state distressing and complain about it. Others, however, accept the situation with resignation, relief, and at times defiance or triumph, so that it is the analyst who has to carry the despair associated with the failure to make contact. Sometimes the retreat is experienced as a cruel place and the deadly nature of the situation is recognized by the patient, but more often the retreat is idealized and represented as a pleasant and even ideal haven. Whether idealized or persecutory, it is clung to as preferable to even worse states which the patient is convinced are the only alternatives. In most patients some movement is observable as they cautiously emerge from the retreat only to return again when things go wrong. In some cases true development is possible in these periods of emergence, and the patient is gradually able to lessen his propensity to withdraw.

In others withdrawal is more prolonged, and if emergence does take place the gains achieved are transitory and the patient returns to his previous state in a negative therapeutic reaction. Typically, an equilibrium is reached in which the patient uses the retreat to remain relatively free from anxiety but at the cost of an almost complete standstill in development. The situation is complicated by the fact that the analyst is used as part of the defensive organization and is sometimes so subtly invited to join in that he does not realize that the analysis itself has been converted into a retreat. The analyst is often under great pressure, and his frustration may lead him to despair or to mount a usually futile effort to overcome what are perceived as the patient's stubborn defences.

All gradations of dependence on the retreat are found clinically, from the completely stuck patient at one extreme to those who use the retreat in a transient and discretionary way at the other. The range and pervasiveness of the retreat may also vary, and some patients are able to develop and sustain adequate relationships in some areas but remain stuck in other aspects of their lives. One of the points I will emphasize throughout this book is that change is possible even in the analysis of very stuck patients. If the analyst is able to persevere and survive the pressure he is put under, he and the patient can gradually come to gain some insight into the operation of the organization and to loosen the grip and the range of its operation.

One of the features of the retreat which emerges most clearly in perverse, psychotic, and borderline patients is the way the avoidance of contact with the analyst is at the same time an avoidance of contact with reality. The retreat then serves as an area of the mind where reality does not have to be faced, where phantasy and omnipotence can exist unchecked and where anything is permitted. This feature is often what makes the retreat so attractive to the patient and commonly involves the use of perverse or psychotic mechanisms.

I am impressed by the power of the system of defences which one can observe operating in these stuck analyses. Sometimes they are so successful that the patient is protected from anxiety, and no difficulty arises as long as the system remains unchallenged. Others remain stuck in the retreat despite the evident suffering it brings, which may be chronic and sustained or masochistic and addictive. In all of these, however, the patient is threatened by the possibility of change and, if provoked, may respond with a more profound withdrawal.

These situations are of great theoretical interest but my own concern is primarily clinical, and this means that my central preoccupation is with the way organizations function in individual patients in individual sessions during an analysis. Here it is important to recognize that the analyst is never able to be an uninvolved observer since he is always to a greater or lesser degree enlisted to participate in enactments in the transference (Sandler 1976; Sandler and Sandler 1978; Joseph 1989). In developing these ideas in the area of pathological organizations I have taken note of the way the patient will use the analyst to help create a sanctuary into which he can retreat. I have been most concerned to follow the situation in the fine grain of the session and to describe how the patient makes moves to emerge from the sanctuary only to retreat again when he confronts anxieties he cannot or will not bear.

It was the highly organized nature of the process which struck me and which led me to use the term 'pathological organization' to describe the internal configuration of defences. The clinical picture itself has become familiar to most working analysts and has been described in various terms by a number of writers whose work is reviewed later in the book. Abraham's (1919, 1924) study of narcissistic resistance and Reich's (1933) work on 'character armour' are early examples. Riviere (1936) spoke about a highly organized system of defences, and Rosenfeld (1964, 1971a) described the operation of destructive narcissism. Segal (1972), O'Shaughnessy (1981), Riesenberg-Malcolm (1981), and Joseph (1982, 1983) have also described patients caught up in powerful defensive systems. This and other similar work has been concerned with patients in extreme situations which can be thought of in relation to those ultimate obstacles to change which Freud addressed in 'Analysis terminable and interminable' (1937). Freud linked these deepest obstacles to change to the operation of the death instinct and, in my view, pathological organizations have a particular role to play in the universal problem of dealing with primitive destructiveness. This affects the individual in profound ways, whether it arises from external or internal sources. Traumatic experiences with violence or neglect in the environment leads to the internalization of violent disturbed objects which at the same time serve as suitable receptacles for the projection of the individual's own destructiveness.

It is not necessary to resolve controversial issues about the death instinct to recognize that there is often something very deadly and self-destructive in the individual's make-up which threatens his integrity unless it is adequately contained. In my view, defensive organizations serve to bind, to neutralize, and to control primitive destructiveness whatever its source, and are a universal feature of the defensive make-up of all individuals. Moreover, in some patients where problems related to destructiveness are particularly prominent, the organization comes to dominate the psyche, and it is these cases which allow its mode of operation to be most readily appreciated.

Once recognized, similar if less disturbing versions can be identified in neurotic and normal individuals.

It is not clear if these methods of dealing with the destructiveness are ever really successful. Certainly, the forms of organization we usually observe tend to function as a kind of compromise and are as much an expression of the destructiveness as a defence against it. Because of this compromise they are always pathological, even though they may serve an adaptive purpose and provide an area of relief and transient protection. Pathological organizations stultify the personality, prevent contact with reality, and ensure that growth and development are interfered with. In normal individuals they are brought into play when anxiety exceeds tolerable limits and are relinquished once more when the crisis is over. Nevertheless, they remain potentially available and can serve to take the patient out of contact and give rise to a stuck period of analysis if the analytic work touches on issues at the edge of what is tolerable. In the more disturbed patient they come to dominate the personality and the patient is to a greater or lesser degree caught in their grip.

The distinction between psychotic and non-psychotic parts of the personality introduced by Bion (1957) can help to differentiate the types of organization which arise in severely disturbed patients from those which exist in neurotic and normal patients, and this is discussed in Chapter 6, where a psychotic organization is described. In psychotic and borderline patients, the organization dominates the personality, where it is used to patch up damaged parts of the ego and as a result is indispensable to the psychotic part of the personality. The non-psychotic personality is less likely to make destructive attacks on its own mind, and since the situation is less desperate a more fluid type of alternation between projective and introjective processes can occur. Despite these differences there are many elements which pathological organizations of the personality in different types of patient have in common and which come to the fore when the patient is under pressure. If analytic work attempts to help the patient deal with problems at the limit of his capacity, difficult areas are raised even in patients who normally function relatively well, and in these situations the patient is likely to make use of a retreat to which he may in normal circumstances only rarely resort.

Even in normal and neurotic patients when the retreat is often represented as a space which occurs naturally or is provided by the environment, it can be seen to arise from the operation of powerful systems of defences. Occasionally patients themselves recognize how they create the retreat, and may even be able to identify the way it serves as a defence. Mostly, however, the description in terms of defences represents the analyst's point of view and forms part of the

5

analyst's theoretical approach. I have found a close examination of the object relations as they emerge in the transference to be particularly helpful in revealing some of the basic mechanisms which are involved in the workings of a pathological organization. To understand the details of their structure it is necessary to know something about the operation of primitive mechanisms of defence, and in particular about projective identification, which is such a central concept in modern Kleinian psychoanalysis. These are discussed later in the book, and at this point it will suffice to recognize that projective identification leads to a narcissistic type of object relationship similar to that which Freud described perhaps most clearly in his paper on Leonardo (1910). In the most straightforward type of projective identification a part of the self is split off and projected into an object, where it is attributed to the object and the fact that it belongs to the self is denied. The object relationship which results is then not with a person truly seen as separate, but with the self projected into another person and related to as if it were someone else. This is the position of the mythical Narcissus, who fell in love with a strange youth he did not consciously connect with himself. It is also true of Leonardo, who projected his infantile self into his apprentices and looked after them in the way he wished his mother had looked after him (Freud 1910).

A narcissistic type of object relationship based on projective identi-fication is certainly a central aspect of pathological organizations, but this is not in itself sufficient to explain the enormous power and resistance to change which they demonstrate. Moreover, projective identification is not in itself a pathological mechanism and indeed forms the basis of all empathic communication. We project into others to understand better what it feels like to be in their shoes, and an inability or reluctance to do this profoundly affects object relations. However, it is essential to normal mental function to be able to use projective identification in a flexible and reversible way and thus to be able to withdraw projections and to observe and interact with others from a position firmly based in our own identity.

In many pathological states such reversibility is obstructed and the patient is unable to regain parts of the self lost through projective identification, and consequently loses touch with aspects of his person-ality which permanently reside in objects with whom they become identified. Any attribute such as intelligence, warmth, masculinity, aggression, and so on can be projected and disowned in this way and, when reversibility is blocked, results in a depletion of the ego, which no longer has access to the lost parts of the self. At the same time, the object is distorted by having attributed to it the split-off and denied parts of the self.

The study of pathological organizations reported in this book has led me to postulate further complexities of structure. The kind of defensive situation just outlined can arise as a result of normal splitting in which the object is seen as either good or bad and the individual tries to get the help of the good to protect him from the bad. It is clear, as Klein herself emphasized (1952), that such splitting of the object is always accompanied by a corresponding split in the ego, and it is a good part of the self in a relationship with a good object which is kept separate from a bad part of the self in relation to a bad object. If the split is successfully maintained, the good and bad are kept so separate that no interaction between them takes place, but if it threatens to break down, the individual may try to preserve his equilibrium by turning to the protection of the good object and good parts of the self against the bad object and against bad parts of the self. If such measures also fail to maintain an equilibrium, even more drastic means may be resorted to.

For example, pathological splitting with a fragmentation of the self and of the object and their expulsion in a more violent and primitive form of projective identification may take place (Bion 1957). Pathological organizations may then evolve to collect the fragments, and the result may once again give the impression of a protective good object kept separate from bad ones. Now, however, what appears as a relatively straightforward split between good and bad is in fact the result of a splitting of the personality into several elements, each projected into objects and reassembled in a manner which simulates the containing function of an object. The organization may present itself as a good object protecting the individual from destructive attacks, but in fact its structure is made up of good and bad elements derived from the self and from the objects which have been projected into and used as building blocks for the resultant extremely complex organization. In my view, the dependent self which is dominated by the organization may also be complex and not as innocent a victim as may first appear. It is not only the building blocks of the organization which need to be understood but the manner in which they are assembled and held together, because the dependent part of the self, and the analyst too, may become caught up and trapped in the tyrannical and cruel object relations which keep the system intact.

In later chapters I will try to show how in pathological organizations of the personality projective identification is not confined to a single object, but, instead, groups of objects are used which are themselves in a relationship. These objects, usually in fact part-objects, are constructed out of experiences with people found in the patient's early environment. The fantastic figures of the patient's inner world are sometimes based on actual experiences with bad objects and sometimes represent distortions and misrepresentations of early experience. Trauma and deprivation in the patient's history have a profound effect on the creation of pathological organizations of the personality, even though it may not be possible to know how much internal and external factors contributed. What becomes apparent in the here and now of the analysis is that the objects, whether they are chosen from those which pre-exist in the environment or created by the individual, are used for specific defensive purposes, in particular to bind destructive elements in the personality.

I have argued that a central function of pathological organizations of the personality is to contain and neutralize these primitive destructive impulses, and in order to deal with these the patient selects destructive objects into which he can project destructive parts of the self. As Rosenfeld (1971a), Meltzer (1968) and others have described, these objects are often assembled into a 'gang' which is held together by cruel and violent means. These powerfully structured groups of individuals are represented unconsciously in the patient's inner world and appear in dreams as an inter-personal version of the retreat. The place of safety is provided by the group who offer protection from both persecution and guilt as long as the patient does not threaten the domination of the gang. The result of these operations is to create a complex network of object relations, each object containing split-off parts of the self and the group held together in complex ways characteristic of a particular organization. The organization 'contains' the anxiety by offering itself as a protector, and it does so in a perverse way very different from that seen in the case of normal containment, such as that described by Bion, to take place between a normal mother and her baby (Bion 1962a, 1963).

This formulation illustrates the extent to which the organization can become personified. In part this is a result of its evolution in early infancy, when many aspects of nature are experienced by the child as arising from the actions of people. In part, however, it results from the way the inner world remains one peopled by objects in relationships with each other as well as with the subject. No sanctuary is secure unless it is also sanctioned and protected by the social group to which it belongs. Sometimes it is possible to get information about deeper phantasies in which psychic retreats appear as spaces inside objects or part-objects. There may be phantasies of retreating to the mother's womb, anus, or breast, sometimes experienced as a desirable but forbidden place.

One of the major consequences of such a structure is that it is very difficult for the individual to risk a confrontation with these objects and repudiate their methods and aims. As a result, the reversibility of projective identification is interfered with. I will argue later that this reversibility is established through a successful working through of mourning. The process of regaining parts of the self lost through projective identification involves facing the reality of what belongs to the object and what belongs to the self, and this is established most clearly through the experience of loss. It is in the process of mourning that parts of the self are regained, and this achievement may require much working through. Thus a true internalization of the object can only be achieved if it is relinquished as an external object. It can then be internalized as separate from the self and in this state can be identified with in a flexible and reversible way. The development of symbolic function assists this process and allows the individual to identify with aspects of the object rather than its concrete totality.

When containment is provided by an organization of objects rather than by a single object it is very difficult for projective identification to be reversed. It is not possible to let any single object go, mourn it, and, in the process, withdraw projections from it, because it does not operate in isolation but has powerful links which bind it to other members of the organization. These links are often ruthlessly maintained, with the primary aim of keeping the organization intact. In fact, the individuals are often experienced as bound inextricably to each other and the containment is felt to be provided by a group of objects treated as if it were a single object; namely, the organization.

To withdraw projections from one of the objects means that reality has to be faced in the area of that particular object relationship and then what belongs to the object and what belongs to the self must be differentiated so that the projection can be separated off and returned to the self. Even if defences operate singly this may be difficult, but when the object relations are part of a complex organization the inter-relationships ensure that the difficulty is extreme. The patient then feels trapped in an omnipotent organization from which there is no escape. If the analyst recognizes the omnipotence he or she is less likely to try to confront or combat the organization head-on. Such recognition, in my view, helps both analyst and patient to live with the omnipotence without either giving in to it or aggressively confronting it. If it can be recognized as one of the facts of life making up the reality of the patient's inner world, then gradually it may become possible to understand it better and as a result to reduce the hold it has on the personality.

I have emphasized how pathological organizations of the personality can result in a stuck patient in a stuck analysis, who may be so hidden from contact that it is difficult for the analyst to reach him. In other patients a similar overall situation results not so much from the lack of contact, movement, and development as from the fact that any development which does occur is quickly, and sometimes totally, reversed. Once this is recognized it is often possible to see that similar, more subtle movements are discernible even in the most apparently stuck patient. As a result a more detailed description becomes possible, which involves following the patient as he makes tentative, sometimes almost imperceptible, moves towards contact with the analyst, only to retreat once more as he confronts anxiety. As the patient begins to emerge from the protection of the organization the ready availability of the shelter as a source of relief of anxiety and pain makes retreat a convenient option, and sometimes the experience of contact is so dreaded that withdrawal is immediate. Nevertheless, if this moment of contact is registered by the analyst and interpreted, the patient can sometimes gain an insight into his dread of contact, feel supported by the analyst, and as a result may gradually extend his ability to tolerate it.

If the patient feels the analyst understands the nature of the anxieties which confront him as he begins to emerge from his retreat, he is more likely to feel supported and thus take further steps away from his dependence on the pathological organization of the personality. Here an important distinction exists between the anxieties of the paranoid-schizoid and those of the depressive positions as described by Klein (1946, 1952), and pathological organizations of the personality serve to protect the patient against both sets of anxieties (Steiner 1979, 1987). This point of view suggests that it is important not only to describe the mental mechanisms which operate at any particular moment but also to discuss their function: that is, not only what is happening but why it is happening – in this instance to try to understand what it is that the patient fears would result if he emerged from the retreat. If the minute movements are attended to, a transient and briefly bearable 'taste' of the anxiety which is experienced on emergence from the retreat can be registered by the patient and interpreted by the analyst as it becomes observable. This can allow the function of the defence to be identified and investigated. Some patients depend on the organization to protect them from primitive states of fragmentation and persecution, and they fear that states of extreme anxiety would overwhelm them if they were to emerge from the retreat. Others have been able to develop a greater degree of integration but are unable to face the depressive pain and guilt which arise as contact with internal and external reality increases. In either case, emergence to make contact with the analyst may lead to a rapid withdrawal to the retreat and an attempt to regain the previously held equilibrium.

Melanie Klein (1952) described the paranoid–schizoid and depressive positions in terms of a grouping of defences, and a pattern of anxieties and other emotions. Each is characterized also by typical

10

mental structures and by typical forms of object relationship, both internal and external. It is in relationship to these positions that pathological organizations can most readily be understood, and indeed the retreat can also be thought of as a position with its own grouping of anxieties, its pattern of defences, its typical object relations and characteristic structure. I have previously referred to it as a 'borderline position' because of its place on the border between the two basic positions (Steiner 1987, 1990a).

The terminology of the positions can be confusing because of the inferred connection to particular types of clinical disorder. Klein had to emphasize that the paranoid–schizoid position did not imply paranoid psychosis in any simple way nor the depressive position, depressive illness. In the same way, the term 'borderline position' is not confined to borderline patients, and although it is true that psychic retreats can be readily observed in borderline states they are also a prominent feature of psychotic patients at one extreme and of normal and neurotic individuals at times of stress, at the other. Klein herself occasionally spoke of a manic position and an obsessional position (Klein 1946), and these more organized defensive states have many features in common with psychic retreats. It is clear that not only the basic two positions but also the borderline position occur in all patients, and the notion of positions can help the analyst to consider where the patient is located at any particular time.

The patient can withdraw to a retreat at a borderline position where he is under the protection of a pathological organization from either of the two basic positions. This theme is elaborated later in the book, where use is made of a triangular equilibrium diagram to illustrate that as the patient emerges from the retreat he may find himself confronted with anxieties from either of the two basic positions.

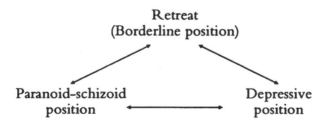

When the analysis is stuck there is very little, if any, movement discernible in this equilibrium, and the patient becomes firmly established in the retreat protected by the pathological organization and only rarely emerges to face either depressive or paranoid–schizoid

11

anxieties. In less stuck situations, which of course occur in patients who may nevertheless be quite ill, and even psychotic, more movement is discernible and shifts occur in which anxieties are at least transiently faced. Here the loss of equilibrium may give rise to severe anxiety and immediate return to the retreat, but it may also enable analytic development to take place.

A striking finding with some examples of a pathological organization of the personality is that the organization is adhered to even when some development has taken place and the need for it no longer appears to be so convincing. It is as if the patient has become accustomed and even addicted to the state of affairs in the retreat and gains a kind of perverse gratification from it. The part of the patient which is in touch with reality is often seduced away by bribes and threats, and the whole organization keeps itself together by creating perverse links between its component members. Indeed, perverse mechanisms play a central role in pathological organizations, particularly in cementing the organization together and underpinning its immovable structure.

A particular type of relationship with reality which is characteristic of retreats plays an important role in preventing the move towards the depressive position which is necessary for development to occur. Freud, in his discussion of fetishism (Freud 1927), described how the patient adopts a stance in which reality is neither fully accepted nor fully disavowed, so that contradictory views are held simultaneously and are reconciled in a variety of ways. In my view, a central aspect of the perverse attitude is reflected in this kind of relation to reality. It is important in *sexual* perversions, where some of the basic 'facts of life', such as the difference between the sexes and between the generations, are simultaneously accepted and disavowed, but it has a more general applicability to any aspect of reality which is difficult to accept. In particular, we see it prominent in the difficult task of facing the reality of ageing and death to which a similarly perverse stance is often taken. A perverse pseudo–acceptance of reality is one of the factors which makes the retreat so attractive for the patient who can keep sufficient contact with reality to appear 'normal' while at the same time evading its most painful aspects.

A second aspect of perversion is seen when the object relations which make up the organization are examined. The links which bind the organization together are often sado–masochistic and involve a cruel type of tyranny in which objects and the patient himself are controlled and bullied in a ruthless way. Sometimes the sadism is obvious, but often the tyranny is idealized and develops a seductive hold on the patient, who appears to become addicted to it, often gaining a masochistic gratification in the process.

12

It is only with long and painful work that the patient begins to feel he has the capacity to say 'no' to the attractive pull of the perversion as alternative sources of help become available. He may then feel less entrapped by the organization and feel he only need turn to its protection at times of particular stress. As the addictive properties lessen he is able to free himself more and face psychic reality. Once this becomes even partially possible, mourning and loss lead to a partial recovery of parts of the self and the dependence on the organization is further loosened. It nevertheless always remains part of the personality where the patient can retreat when reality becomes unbearable. If it is recognized for what it is – namely, an area where perverse relationships and perverse thinking are sanctioned – the patient may accept an occasional need to adopt these methods without idealizing them. The protection of the retreat is then seen to offer a temporary respite from anxiety but no real security and no opportunity for development. Like other elements in the inner world, it can then be viewed more realistically and the patient can come to terms with it.

This preliminary outline will be expanded in the following chapters. It is clear that a psychic retreat can be conceptualized in a variety of different ways. First, it can be viewed spatially as an area of safety to which the patient withdraws, and second, this area can be seen to depend on the operation of a pathological organization of the personality. The organization itself can be seen as a highly structured system of defences and also as a tightly organized network of object relations. The retreat may also be usefully related to the paranoid–schizoid and depressive positions and can then be seen to function as a third position to which the patient can withdraw from the anxieties of either of the former. Finally, the perverse nature of the retreat can be viewed from the point of view of the patient's relationship with reality on the one hand and in terms of the sado–masochistic type of object relationships found, on the other.

Patients who find themselves trapped in a psychic retreat present formidable technical problems for the analyst. He has to struggle to cope with a patient who is out of contact and an analysis which seems to be getting nowhere for very long periods. The analyst also has to struggle with his own propensity both to fit in and collude with the organization on the one hand and to withdraw into his own defensive retreat, on the other. If the analyst comes to understand some of the processes better, he is more able to recognize the patient's situation and to be available at those times when the patient does emerge to make contact possible.

2

Psychic retreats: a clinical illustration[1]

In this chapter I will present clinical material from a patient (Mrs A) in a relatively stuck analysis in order to illustrate the function of psychic retreats in the to and fro of analytic work. One of the chief technical problems with this patient was her silence, which often extended for most of the session and indeed for several sessions. Despite this there were periods when she was more free, and she was sometimes able to bring dreams and other material which helped me to understand her experience in the stuck periods. Both in her everyday life and in the sessions she was able to make transient contact which enabled some progress to occur, but it was frequently cut short in an abrupt and violent way.

I will illustrate how it was possible to observe a withdrawal to a refuge where the patient was relatively free from anxiety but where development was minimal. The withdrawal protected the patient from contact and the history suggested that it had functioned in that way for many years. Shortly before she began analysis the defensive organization which gave rise to the retreat had broken down and periods of panic and persecution ensued which led her to seek treatment. Once in analysis she used the treatment and the relationship with the analyst to re-create the retreat. This provided relief from the panic but re-established the rigid defensive organization.

The patient's silence seemed to mark those periods when she retreated out of contact. For a long time it was idealized and served as a position of strength from which she could mock and denigrate the analysis. She effectively projected the desire to make contact into me and would watch as I struggled with my uncertainty about how to

---

1 This chapter is based on some of the ideas and the clinical material previously published in Steiner (1987).

react. It seemed wrong for me to remain silent, but attempts to reach her were mostly ineffective. If I was patient I could make a tentative contact from time to time and was then sometimes able to follow the patient and stay in touch, until something would go wrong and she would abruptly withdraw.

Although the withdrawal appeared to break contact with the analyst, a closer consideration of what happened revealed that the withdrawal in fact established a different type of interaction which was by no means less intense. This pathological type of contact involved an intense sado–masochistic interaction between patient and analyst and was characteristic of the way she functioned in the retreat. Although in many ways distressing and even persecuting to her, it served to protect the patient from 'real contact' which would put her in touch with psychic reality.

The patient's dreams and reports of her phantasy life provided information about the nature of the retreat she withdrew to and revealed its protective function. It was sometimes possible to follow the movements in the session and to link these with the images she brought in dreams and other material. This gave an idea of the nature of the anxiety she faced, which varied. For much of the analysis, especially in the beginning, the anxiety was that associated with panic, frag-mentation, depersonalization, and persecution. Later, however, there were hints that she also feared depressive pain. The retreat then served to avoid contact with loss, guilt, and other anxieties associated with the depressive position.

Sometimes she gave the impression that the retreat was held onto and used for reasons other than protection from anxiety and pain. There was often a perverse flavour to the interaction, and cruelty was prominent at these times. There was also an addictive quality, as if the retreat was being used to give gratification, and any progress that had been made was kept secret in order that adherence to the retreat could be justified.

The patient was often difficult to understand, and it was not easy to assess the nature of her anxiety or to know whether I was working well or badly; this was particularly so at those times when she would make contact and then abruptly withdraw as if she had been shocked or hurt by me.

History

The patient was an attractive, recently married woman in her twenties who had dropped out of university and who tended to develop withdrawn states when she would take to her bed and do nothing except read novels endlessly. When she was still a baby, her family had escaped from a country where they experienced political persecution. They were occasionally able to return to visit her grandmother, and these visits and the border crossings they entailed were especially anxious times for her.

She sought treatment because of attacks of incapacitating anxiety, at first associated with major decisions such as whether she should stay in England, or whether she should let her future husband move into her flat when, at that time, he did not intend to marry her. They would also occur when she got involved in long discussions on existential themes, which resulted in panic when she realized that she saw no meaning in life. She would find herself trembling, would feel her surroundings recede and become distant, and found that she could not make contact with people because a diffuse barrier came between them. When her husband agreed to marry her the anxiety lessened but would reappear periodically – for example, once when she lost a locket containing a piece of his hair. In addition, she suffered from a specific fear of being poisoned from tinned food which she would become convinced had been contaminated. Even between anxiety attacks she was preoccupied with pollution and poisoning, and had terrifying dreams in which, for example, radioactivity produced a kind of living death and people became automata. A fascination with deadness and aridity was linked to a preoccupation with the Sahara Desert which she had visited and to which she planned to return on an expedition when her treatment was over.

Behaviour in the sessions

A central feature of the analysis was the fact that she was a silent patient – in fact, often silent for the greater part of the session for months on end. She would begin with a long silence or a comment such as, 'Nothing has happened', or 'It is going to be another silent session'. Occasionally she would give an explanation and, for example, say, 'I sort things out into what I could say and what I couldn't say, and the things I could say are not worth saying'. Very often there was a mocking, teasing quality, usually accompanied by a sulky little girl voice. 'I felt totally misunderstood yesterday and I am not going to say anything today, so there!' Or she might admit that she said to herself, 'Don't show anything to him unless you have thought it all out so he cannot find fault with it', or 'Don't say anything to him unless you are sure you can win the argument'. The silence might turn into a game in

16

which she would alternate between starting a session herself or making me start, or she might gamble on how long she would have to wait before I spoke. During the silence she often thought of herself as sunbathing on a desert island, and she acknowledged that she enjoyed these games and their accompanying fantasies. The most prominent mood was of a smiling indifference, a kind of nonchalance and a playful lack of concern in which the difficulties of the analysis and indeed the realities of life going on around her were *my* problem. This sometimes made me feel exploited and put upon as if I had colluded with the notion that I should care more about her analysis than she did. At other times I was provoked to interpret her lack of concern in a critical way, as if I was trying to persuade her to become more caring because I was unwilling to take on the responsibility.

At the same time there was a deadly seriousness about her analysis, and she was rarely late and almost never missed a session. On one occasion, when I had let a silence go on for longer than usual, she began to weep silently, and when I asked her what she was thinking I was told a tragic story about a girl who had taken an overdose and was left to die because nobody came until it was too late.

As she lay on the couch, the patient would move her hands restlessly and incessantly. She would pick at her fingernails in a jerky and irritating way, or pull threads out of a bandage or out of her clothing or play with her sleeve or her buttons. For a time she found it hard to resist picking at the wallpaper next to the couch, where there was a small raised piece at an edge which she longed to pull off. Most often she played with her long hair, pulling down a bunch as if milking it, teasing out individual hairs, making patterns with them, twisting them and then milking them free again. I was reminded of Freud's statement in the Dora case that, 'no mortal can keep a secret. If his lips are silent, he chatters with his finger tips' (1905a), but for the most part I could not understand the factors behind her silence or the meaning of the hand movements.

She would say that she had a large number of thoughts which she could not string together, and this suggested a fragmentation of her thoughts. However, it was also clear that something active, teasing, and pleasurable was going on. The overall atmosphere was one of long periods of deadness and aridity in which no development was discernible.

On the basis of the history and the description of the patient's general behaviour it is possible to put forward the idea that she retreated to a refuge which protected her from contact and which was represented by her image of a desert island where she could sunbathe and leave the responsibility for the analysis to me. The feeling of aridity and deadness associated with this state was well represented by the preoccupation with sand and her love of deserts, and it was important to her that she should learn to cope with conditions where life could barely survive.

Sometimes the refuge appeared to break down and the anxiety emerged in the form of attacks of panic. This was the case before the analysis began, and the initial rapid improvement as she began treatment resulted from the re-establishment of a refuge, now using the analyst and the analysis as part of the defensive organization. For the most part the panic appeared to involve a fear of disintegration or a paranoid fear of being poisoned. Later, as we shall see, the refuge was utilized as a protection against depressive feelings as well.

Material from a session

She began a session some two years into the analysis, by hunting in her bag for her cheque which she eventually gave me, and which I noticed she had filled in wrongly, forgetting the figures.

She then spoke after only a short silence to tell me a dream in which she had invited a young couple for a meal and then realized that she had run out of something, probably wine or food. Her husband and the friends went out to get the provisions while she waited at home. When they returned they brought the girl back on a stretcher and explained that she had been cut through at the waist and had no lower half. The girl was not upset but smiled and later went off on crutches. The patient asked her husband to take her to show her where it had happened. He did this and explained how a car had hit her from behind and cut her in two.

It was a relief to have a dream instead of the silence, and I interpreted that the dream itself might represent provisions for the analysis, as if she realized that we had run out of material to work with. The girl in the dream had been violently attacked when she went out for the provisions, and I suggested that she might be afraid that something similar would happen to her if she brought material for analysis. Perhaps, I added, she was less afraid of being attacked now and could express a wish to understand these fears, represented in the dream by the request to find out how the accident had happened.

She was attentive and nodded as if she understood what I meant, and this led me to go on a little later and try to link the dream with her experience at the beginning of the session when she was hunting for her cheque. I suggested that she might be divided in her feelings about paying me, having brought the cheque and then losing it in her handbag, and also by filling it in incompletely.

There was a sharp change of mood and the patient became flippant, saying that if that was the case she could put it right immediately because she had a pen with her, and she did not want me to have anything I could use in evidence against her. It felt as if the contact with her had been abruptly cut off. She now seemed to feel that I had caught her out and was making a fuss, using her mistake with the cheque to put pressure on her to admit her ambivalence and to talk about her feelings. A mistake which she had not noticed left her feeling dangerously out of control, and she had to attack the mood of co-operation and correct the mistake as quickly as possible. The mood in the earlier part of the session had, however, given a feeling of contact, and I think it did represent a move out of the protection of the retreat. This, however, stimulated a violent attack when I went too far or perhaps too fast, to link it up with something actual which had happened in the session.

The violence of the break in contact was striking, just as had been the violence to the girl in the dream. She had emerged to make contact in order to get provisions, indicating an admission that she felt the lack of something and wanted something for herself and her guests. But something went wrong and she reverted to a state of mind in which she was cut in two just as the girl had been in the dream. In my interpretations I linked the way that she was cut off from her feelings in the session with the indifferent, smiling, flippant lack of concern of the girl in her dream who smiled and did not mind being cut in two.

There was also an innuendo that I was more concerned with my cheque than with her needs, so that she quickly took out her pen as if she had to satisfy my greed. This led me to doubt my motives and made me feel that I had let her down and that I had changed from someone who understood her anxiety about being attacked into someone felt to be attacking her by pointing out her mistake in the cheque. It may also be possible that she unconsciously set things up so that I would both make contact with her in response to her dream and also that I would 'spoil' this contact by appearing to criticize her for the faulty cheque. The result was just that described in the dream, namely, that the attack was directed against the relationship with me and against any part of her which had a desire to cooperate with the analytic work by bringing material and by acknowledging her ambivalence and attempting to understand it. At first, evidence for an interest in the analysis of the dream and in the desire to understand her state of mind was discernible, which I thought was represented in the dream by her wish to understand where and how the accident to her friend had happened. Subsequently, this disappeared from view and the desire to understand resided in the analyst, and she directed her endeavours to keeping me at bay.

Progress of the analysis

Acknowledging progress was particularly difficult and usually led to such violent attacks that she seldom admitted any improvement in our working relationship or, indeed, in her life in general. It was only in passing that I heard, over the next few months, that she had applied to an art school for which she was preparing a portfolio, and that she was taking driving lessons. She did, however, mention that her husband was installing central heating, and that although she was reluctant to leave her art work, she had somewhat grudgingly agreed to help him. She had become quite involved and interested in this work, and had admitted that when she did bring herself to help she found it satisfying. 'I have become quite an expert on radiators and boilers,' she said. This seemed to correspond to a warmer atmosphere which had begun to develop in her sessions, although the grudging, sulky and sensitive mood had by no means completely lifted.

She then failed to turn up for three sessions, and because this was so unusual I telephoned her to enquire what had happened. She explained that while working on the central heating she had dropped a radiator on her toe and that she had tried to ring me at her session time, but I had failed to answer – in fact, because my telephone bell had inadvertently been turned off.

Material from a second session

On her return she could admit that not only her toe but her feelings had been hurt by my failure to be available, and she had once more taken to her bed and her novels.

She then described a dream in which a girl had died of a mysterious illness and she had been summoned by the girl's parents to talk to them. She did not know what to say, and was told that it did not matter, as if they saw that she was upset and were being careful not to make her cry. She added, 'You can say, "How nice", when something good happens but . . . if something bad has happened . . .'. In the dream the room to which she had been summoned contained bookshelves and a coal stove which she was able to link to bookshelves in a children's home where she had been left as an infant.

20

She idealized her memories of this home – in particular, the beautiful dolls there – but in fact said that she had been left there while the family went on holiday with her younger brother and on their return she refused to recognize her mother and became so ill that she was unable to leave the home for a further two weeks.

A further association then emerged to a waiting room on the frontier when the family had been stopped after a visit to her grandmother. Her mother had on this occasion been taken off the train by border guards to have some irregularity in her passport checked, and the family waited for her in a room with bookshelves and a coal stove.

I was able to interpret that elements in the dream reflected her feeling that when I did not answer the telephone, a tragic event like a death from a mysterious illness had occurred, and that when I had telephoned her, it felt as if I had summoned her back to the analysis to ask her to explain her reaction. I think the analytic work represented by the installing of central heating had put her more in touch with her feelings, and the associations to the dream confirmed that horrific memories were revived of times when she feared she might lose her mother.

Discussion

If we look back at the fragment of material from the first session, it is possible to see how a degree of contact was allowed as she followed my analysis of the dream in which going out for food was linked to getting material for the analysis. She could even recognize that the dream showed how afraid she was of a violent attack and that she wanted to be shown how and where it happened. Then, the contact was suddenly and violently broken, as I connected the whole situation to the fact that she had left the numbers out when she wrote the cheque. The contact was replaced with the flippant superiority which came from the protection of her refuge and I was quickly left isolated and rejected. The implication was that I had done something terrible and that she had to protect herself from the trauma I had created. The climate was a persecutory one and as she retreated one got a glimpse of a panicky feeling which made contact too terrifying to sustain. While at first she could appreciate that she had paranoid fears and make contact with me as someone who could help her with them, we could not prevent them from being enacted in the session, and when this happened she felt obliged to return to the refuge.

In the second session the retreat to the refuge followed my failure to answer her telephone call, and the atmosphere at this time was very different. Progress in the analysis had occurred even though it was rarely admitted, and the work on the central heating in cooperation with her husband was reflected by a greater warmth in the sessions. Then, when I failed to answer her telephone call, she was dismayed. She had little capacity to sustain loss, and just as a warmer relationship was developing and she was able to mobilize a bit more contact she found herself betrayed. It is understandable that she would be seduced back into her refuge from which she could approach me with flippancy and a lack of concern. She took to her bed and resumed the endless reading of novels which had been a feature of her behaviour before the analysis began. At the same time she was less panicky, and the pain connected with the contact appeared more to do with loss and anxiety about loss. Her dream connected with memories of being left, and, later, with the border crossings when she must have been terrified of losing her mother. The refuge was at this stage represented by the room on the border which had the coal stove and bookshelves and in the dream was connected with the family who had lost a daughter. Nevertheless, it was still a place which was idealized and used to avoid contact. She could retreat to a state of mind when her feelings were hurt and which kept her away from the analysis. It is hard to know how long she might have stayed in bed if I had not telephoned her. She did seem to be relieved by the telephone call and she responded to it and was able to resume analytic work although she remained very sensitive and easily hurt.

The refuge appeared in the patient's material in spatial terms, as a place to which she could retreat and gain safety. Later I will show how it can also be represented in terms of complex object relationships which I call a pathological organization of the personality. Equally, it can be thought to arise from the operation of primitive defence mechanisms which are intertwined to make up a defensive system. These various ways of describing the retreat reflect different aspects of the same clinical phenomena.

The refuge offered the patient an idealized haven from the terrifying situations around her but also appeared to provide other sources of gratification. The perverse flavour was connected with the apparent lack of concern on the part of the patient, and the evident pleasure and power she derived from the self-sufficiency of the retreat. The analyst, by contrast, feels extremely uncomfortable, being asked to carry the concern and yet knowing from his experience with the patient that whatever he does will be unsatisfactory. If I had not telephoned the patient I had the impression that she would not have been able to make the move towards me and we might have had a very long absence or even a breakdown in the analysis. On the other hand, I was also left feeling that telephoning her was a serious error in technique, and I had an uneasy sense of doing something improper as if I had been seduced or was seducing *her* to make her feel she was coming back to the analysis for my benefit and at my summons. It is interesting to observe that it is sometimes the analyst's shortcomings which are exploited to justify a return to the retreat. Here the patient could argue that my failure to answer her telephone call meant that I had let her down and this justified a retreat to her bed and her novels, which could again be idealized as safe and warm. This makes the analyst feel that any lapse on his part can become a stimulus for a perverse triumph.

The importance of the perverse element will be examined in detail in Chapters 8 and 9 but will be discernible in much of the clinical material in this and other chapters. It was a factor in this patient's silence that was associated in her mind with a retreat to an idealized state which she could call her desert island where she could sunbathe free of concern. I thought she had some insight into the way she created these states of mind, and that the safety she found there was illusory while the deadness and aridity she created was real and extremely disabling. She therefore had a true desire to make progress in the analysis and to find within herself creative capacities which could lead to development professionally and to the satisfaction of a long-hidden wish to have children.

Such developments, however, depended on her capacity to withstand destructive attacks which were regularly mounted whenever she approached the depressive position and made contact with her need of objects and her reparative impulses towards them. In fact, some progress gradually became apparent, and she was less often silent and cut off as she acquired more insight into the way she could be threatened and seduced back into a withdrawal whenever contact with reality became difficult. She began and eventually completed her art degree and passed her driving test. She also made better contact with her husband and parents whom she was able to invite and even to appreciate, and she even finally became pregnant. She had very much wanted to have a baby but the pregnancy revived many primitive anxieties and her propensity to withdraw returned. She stopped her analysis soon after, partly for practical reasons, but returned to see me some three years later. At that time she reported that she had two children and that although she had many difficulties with them, she was coping reasonably well. She was pregnant again and wanted to discuss the question of having an abortion. I thought she saw me as someone who had continued to be available if she needed to make contact and that I represented a figure who supported her in difficult times. I said very little in this consultation but I was interested to hear about her progress, and she wrote to me afterwards to say that she had decided against a termination.

I think it is possible to see how the pathological organization protected the patient from both paranoid–schizoid and depressive anxieties. It offered the comforts of withdrawal to a state which was neither fully alive nor quite dead, and yet something close to death, and relatively free of pain and anxiety. This state was idealized even though the patient knew she was cut off and out of touch with her feelings. I think that perverse sources of gratification were prominent and that these helped to keep her addicted to the relief which the refuge brought. The panic attacks represented a breakdown of the defensive organization and a consequent return to the persecutory fragmentation of the paranoid–schizoid position. At other times it was possible to observe a change of attitude which represented a move towards the depressive position, and these could be recognized as constituting analytically meaningful change. She was able, at least temporarily, to relinquish her dependence on the refuge and establish a relationship with me as her analyst. It was evident, however, how precarious this contact was and how easily it could once more be cut off.

3

The paranoid–schizoid and depressive positions[1]

When a pathological organization of the personality breaks down and ceases to function effectively the patient is thrown into a state of anxiety and panic. The patient may himself refer to this state as a 'breakdown', and it is often what drives him to seek treatment. Frequently the anxiety is overwhelming, and he may in desperation turn to his analysis to re-establish the equilibrium he had before his breakdown and to create out of it a retreat similar to that which protected him previously. It may take much analytic work before the patient will once more risk emerging from the retreat to make contact with the analyst and with psychic reality. Other patients reach this point earlier, and some even seek treatment because they feel stuck in the retreat and want to be free of it. In the course of their lives or through analytic work they feel stronger, and they may get a taste of the satisfactions which reality can provide. As they relinquish the protection of the retreat they are brought up against anxieties, and if these are felt to be unbearable they may withdraw once again.

In this chapter I will examine the different types of situation which the patient meets as he emerges from the psychic retreat from the point of view of the anxieties he confronts as he does so. These can be categorized in a number of ways, but perhaps most helpful is that based on the distinction that Melanie Klein made between two basic group-ings of anxieties and defences, the paranoid–schizoid and depressive positions. I will first briefly describe her ideas and then suggest that more recent work enables us to refine these concepts and to subdivide each of the positions. This leads to a continuum of mental states within the positions, each in a dynamic equilibrium with its neighbour. In this

1 Parts of this chapter have previously been published. See Steiner (1990c) and (1992).

way it is possible to describe those situations which are particularly likely to lead to a withdrawal to a psychic retreat.

The two basic positions

Perhaps the most significant difference between the two basic positions is along the dimension of increasing integration which leads to a sense of wholeness, both in the self and in object relations, as the patient moves from the paranoid–schizoid towards the depressive position. Alongside this comes a shift from a preoccupation with the survival of the self to a recognition of dependence on the object and a consequent concern with the state of the object. However, each of the positions can be compared along almost any dimension of mental life, and in particular in terms of characteristic anxieties, defences, mental structures, and types of object relations. Moreover, a variety of other features such as the type of thinking, feeling or phantasying characterizes the positions, and each can be considered to denote 'an attitude of mind, a constellation of conjoint phantasies and relationships to objects with characteristic anxieties and defences' (Joseph 1983).

The paranoid–schizoid position

In the paranoid–schizoid position (Klein 1946; Segal 1964) anxieties of a primitive nature threaten the immature ego and lead to the mobilization of primitive defences. Klein believed that the individual is threatened by sources of destructiveness from within, based on the death instinct, and that these are projected into the object to create the prototype of a hostile object relationship. The infant hates, and fears the hatred of, the bad object, and a persecutory situation develops as a result. In a parallel way, primitive sources of love, based on the life instinct, are projected to create the prototype of a loving object relationship.

In the paranoid–schizoid position these two types of object relationship are kept as separate as possible, and this is achieved by a split in the object which is viewed as excessively good or extremely bad. States of persecution and idealization tend to alternate, and if one is present the other is usually not far away, having been split off and projected. Together with the split in the object the ego is similarly split, and a bad self is kept as separate as possible from a good self.

In the paranoid–schizoid position the chief defences are splitting, projective identification, and idealization, the structure of the ego reflects the split into good and bad selves in relationship with good and bad objects, and object relationships are likewise split. The ego is poorly integrated over time so that there is no memory of a good object when it is lost. Indeed, the loss of the good object is experienced as the presence of a bad object and the idealized situation is replaced by a persecutory one. Similarly in the spatial dimension, self and objects are viewed as being made up of parts of the body such as the breast, face, or hands and are not yet integrated into a whole person.

Paranoid-schizoid defences also have a powerful effect on thinking and symbol formation. Projective identification leads to a confusion between self and object, and this results in a confusion between the symbol and the thing symbolized (Segal 1957). The concrete thinking which arises when symbolization is interfered with leads to an increase in anxiety and in rigidity.

The depressive position

The depressive position (Klein 1935, 1940; Segal 1964) represents an important developmental advance, in which whole objects begin to be recognized and ambivalent impulses become directed towards the primary object. The infant comes to recognize that the breast which frustrates him is the same as the one which gratifies him, and the result of such integration over time is that ambivalence – that is, both hatred and love for the same object – is felt. These changes result from an increased capacity to integrate experiences and lead to a shift in primary concern from the survival of the self to a concern for the object upon which the individual depends. This results in feelings of loss and guilt which enable the sequence of experiences we know as mourning to take place. The consequences include a development of symbolic function and the emergence of reparative capacities which become possible when thinking no longer has to remain concrete.

The equilibrium: P/S ↔ D

Although the paranoid-schizoid position antedates the depressive position and is more primitive developmentally, Klein preferred the term 'position' to Freud's idea of stages of development because it emphasized the dynamic relationship between the two (Klein 1935; Joseph 1983; Segal 1983). A continuous movement between the two positions takes place so that neither dominates with any degree of completeness or permanence. Indeed, it is these fluctuations which we try to follow clinically as we observe periods of integration leading to depressive position functioning, or disintegration and fragmentation resulting in a paranoid–schizoid state. Such fluctuations can take place over months and years as an analysis develops but can also be seen in the fine grain of a session, as moment-to-moment changes. If the patient makes meaningful progress, a gradual shift towards depressive position function is observed, while if he deteriorates we see a reversion to paranoid–schizoid functioning such as occurs in negative therapeutic reactions. These observations led Bion (1963) to suggest that the two positions were in an equilibrium with each other rather like a chemical equilibrium, and he introduced the chemical style of notation P/S ↔ D. This way of putting it emphasizes the dynamic quality and focuses attention on the factors which lead to a shift in one direction or another.

The retreat adds a third position to this basic equilibrium diagram and enables us to follow shifts between the two positions and also between each of them and the retreat. Although clearly quite distinct from the basic two positions, the retreat does function in relation to them as if it were itself a position. Like the paranoid–schizoid and depressive positions it can be thought of as a grouping of anxieties, defences, and object relations, but its structure is marked by the rigidity conferred through the pathological organizations of the personality. Klein herself (1935, 1940) for a time thought of other positions, and described a *manic position* and an *obsessional position* which functioned as defensive organizations. The similarity between the retreat and a position helps the analyst to remember how the state of mind of the patient may shift, sometimes along the base of the triangle in the way Bion envisaged in his equilibrium P/S ↔ D, and sometimes turning to the retreat if the anxieties in either of the two basic positions became excessive.

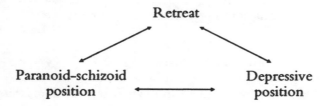

When the analysis is stuck there is very little, if any, movement discernible in this equilibrium, and the patient becomes firmly established in the retreat protected by the pathological organization and only rarely emerges to face either depressive or paranoid–schizoid anxieties. In less stuck situations, which of course occur in patients who may nevertheless be quite ill, and even psychotic, more movement is discernible and shifts occur in which anxieties are at least transiently faced.

The contrast between the two positions has an impressive clarity and simplicity and has proved to be extremely useful. In practice, however, we find defences being deployed in more complex ways, and a deeper understanding of mental mechanisms has led to a distinction between different levels of organization within both the paranoid-schizoid and the depressive positions.

Differentiation within the paranoid-schizoid position

Schematically it is possible to divide the paranoid-schizoid position into a phase involving pathological fragmentation as described by Bion (1957), and one more like that described originally by Klein (Segal 1964) in which normal splitting predominates. These two subdivisions of the paranoid-schizoid position can also be considered to exist in an equilibrium as follows:

Pathological fragmentation   ←——————→   Normal splitting

Normal splitting

Melanie Klein has stressed the importance of normal splitting for healthy development (Klein 1946; Segal 1964). The immature infant has to organize his chaotic experience, and a primitive structure to the ego is provided by a split into good and bad. This reflects a measure of integration that allows a good relationship to a good object to develop by splitting off destructive impulses which are directed towards bad objects. This kind of splitting may be observed clinically, and in infant observation, as an alternation between idealized and persecutory states. If successful, the ego is strengthened to the point where it can tolerate ambivalence, and the split can be lessened to usher in the depressive position. Although idealized, and hence a distortion of reality, the periods of integration, which at this stage take place in relation to good objects, can be seen as precursors of the depressive position.

Pathological fragmentation

Although normal splitting can effectively deal with much of the psychic threat facing the individual, it frequently fails to master all the anxiety, even in relatively healthy individuals, and defences are called on which are more extreme and damaging in their effects. One such situation arises if persecutory anxiety becomes excessive, which may leave the individual feeling that his very survival is threatened. Such a threat may paradoxically lead to further defensive fragmentation, which involves minute splitting and violent projection of the fragments. Bion (1957) has described how this leads to the creation of bizarre objects which intensify the persecution of the patient through experiences of a mad kind.

The result is intense fear, and a sense of chaos and confusion which may be observed clinically in extreme states of panic with depersonalization and derealization, where the patient describes feelings of being in tiny pieces or of being assaulted by strange experiences, sometimes in the form of hallucinations. The individual may yet tolerate such periods of extreme anxiety if the normal split can be maintained so that good experiences can survive. If splitting breaks down, however, the whole personality may be invaded by anxiety, which can result in an intolerable state with catastrophic consequences. Such a breakdown of splitting is particularly threatened if envy is prominent, since destructive attacks are then mounted against good objects, and it is impossible to keep all the destruction split off. A confusional state may then develop which often has particularly unbearable qualities (Klein 1957; Rosenfeld 1950).

Pathological organizations are particularly likely to be deployed to deal with the anxieties which arise in the phase of pathological fragmentation. Minute splitting and fragmentation with catastrophic anxiety in which the self is felt to be splintered and disintegrating may be so unbearable that defensive organizations are needed to create some kind of order out of the chaos. In these desperate states even omnipotent organizations with psychotic characteristics may give relief. Those with experience of general psychiatry will recognize a striking example of this in the case of some patients who are admitted to hospital in a pre-psychotic state. It is possible to observe patients in a 'delusional mood', in which extreme anxiety is accompanied by depersonalization and feelings of ill-defined dread, who may actually appear relieved as the diffuse dread gives way to fixed systematized delusions. Some patients, in fact, visibly calm down and cheer up, as the anxiety and persecution become restricted to the area of the delusional system under the control of a psychotic organization.

Patient A

I will first present some clinical material from a consultation interview with a patient operating at the paranoid-schizoid level in which fears were predominantly those of fragmentation and persecution.

From the beginning of the interview the patient was consumed with anger. His wife had suffered several breakdowns requiring hospital admission, and a social worker had been seeing them as a couple. She had then arranged for his wife to have individual treatment, and the patient was furious and arranged his own referral to the Tavistock Clinic. He was able to say very little about himself, and when I pointed this out he became indignant, saying that he thought it unreasonable for a patient who had problems in communication to be expected to communicate. After several attempts to get through to him which led nowhere I asked for a dream.

He described one in which he met a friend and was offered a lift home on his motorbike. They drove all over London and ended up at the river, which was nowhere near his home. In the dream he got angry and said it would have been quicker to go home by himself.

I interpreted that this was the feeling in the session where I was taking him all over the place but not where he wanted to go. I suggested that he was fed up and wondered why he had come at all. To this he said, 'Very clever.'

When I asked for an early memory he described several vaguely, but when pressed for detail he recalled a time as a small child when someone gave him a glass to drink from. He bit completely through it and ended up with pieces of glass in his mouth. Before that he thought he had been used to flexible plastic cups. I linked this with his rage in the session and his fear that things around him were cracking up. I interpreted that he was afraid I couldn't be flexible like the plastic cup, but might crack up as his wife had done. He was able then to acknowledge his violence and to admit that he hit his wife and also smashed the furniture at home. It remained impossible to work with him, since to be flexible seemed to mean to become completely pliable and allow him to dictate how the session and his treatment should be conducted.

With only the brief contact of a consultation interview it is not possible to describe this patient's defensive organization in any detail, but the arrogant and demanding way he related in the session suggested an organization which held sway over its objects by bullying and threats. When the patient's wife broke down, instead of complying and fitting in with the patient's demands, the organization also threatened

31

to break down and it was this which brought the patient to the consultation. He was not able to cope without it, I think, because he felt that his arrogant and demanding nature was needed to avoid an internal chaos and confusion. He did not know how to cope with his wife's illness, perhaps because it reminded him so vividly of his own, and any relinquishment of his angry omnipotence threatened to expose the chaos and confusion.

Patient B

A 25-year-old artist would become irrationally terrified that his plumbing would leak, that his central heating would break down, that his telephone would be cut off, and so on. He was extremely anxious to start analysis and immediately became very excited, convinced that he was my star patient, and wondered if I was writing a book about him. Very quickly, however, he felt trapped and insisted on keeping a distance by producing breaks in the analysis, which created an atmosphere where I was invited to worry about him and prevent him from leaving. The extent of his claustro–agoraphobic anxieties was illustrated when he went to Italy for a holiday. Because of his country of origin he needed a visa, and although he knew this he had simply neglected to get one. When the immigration officials in Rome told him that he would have to return to London he created such a scene, crying and shouting, that they relented and let him in. Once in the country, however, he became frightened that he wouldn't be allowed out because the officials would see that his passport had not been stamped. He, therefore, managed to cajole his friends to take him to the French border which he crossed in the boot of their car, obtained the necessary visa, and re-entered in the normal way to continue his holiday.

It is clear that he regularly left me to carry the worry and concern for him, and this became particularly so when he behaved in a similar way when he took a holiday to the Soviet Union. This time he found that his visa did not correctly match the departure date and he simply took a pen and altered it. He did return safely and soon after had the following dream.

He was in a Moscow hotel with a homosexual friend and wanted to masturbate with him. Two lady guides, however, refused to leave the room and indeed were proud of their work and of the hotel, even arranging to serve excellent meals in the room. The patient complained about this because he felt trapped, not even being allowed to go to the restaurant, and even began to suspect that the guides had connections with the KGB.

The panic which constantly afflicted this patient was basically that which resulted when things got out of control. His defensive organization was an attempt to deal with this chaotic anxiety by omnipotent methods in which he would force himself into his objects and then feel claustrophobic and have to escape in great anxiety. His dream of the Soviet Union did seem to contain a representation of a good object in the form of the two lady guides, perhaps representing the analysis, who served excellent meals, but his basic reaction to them was persecutory and he complained that he was imprisoned and not allowed to go to the restaurant. What the guides did was to interfere with his homosexual activity by their presence, and I think this is what the analysis was beginning to do. Although he did seem to appreciate what he was offered in the analysis, he could not risk losing the protection of the pathological organizations of the personality. Progress and particularly meaningful contact led to violent negative therapeutic reactions associated with a return to promiscuous homosexuality.

In both these patients anxiety threatened when the organization broke down and failed to provide an adequate retreat. The breakdown of the organization is what led them to seek treatment, which they hoped would re-establish their previous equilibrium. Although it interfered with development and created enormous problems for them, the retreat did seem to protect them from paranoid-schizoid fragmentation, and any emergence from it to make contact with the analyst was resisted.

Differentiation within the depressive position

Splitting is not restricted to the paranoid-schizoid position (Klein 1935), and is resorted to again when the good object has been internalized as a whole object and ambivalent impulses towards it lead to depressive states in which the object is felt to be damaged, dying, or dead and 'casts its shadow on the ego' (Freud 1917). Attempts to possess and preserve the good object are part of the depressive position and lead to a renewal of splitting, this time to prevent the loss of the good object and to protect it from attacks.

The aim in this phase of the depressive position is to deny the reality of the loss of the object, and this state of mind is similar to that of the bereaved person in the early stages of mourning. In mourning it appears as a normal stage which needs to be passed through before the subsequent experience of acknowledgement of the loss can take place.

An important mechanism deployed in this denial is a type of projective identification which leads to possession of the object by identifying

33

with it. Freud himself (1941) suggested that the notion of 'having an object' arises later than the more primitive one of 'being the object'. He wrote, 'Example: the breast. "The breast is part of me, I am the breast." Only later: "I have it" — that is, "I am not it".' Moreover, in this brief note he adds that after a loss 'having' relapses to 'being'.

A critical point in the depressive position arises when the task of relinquishing control over the object has to be faced. The earlier trend, which aims at possessing the object and denying reality, has to be reversed if the depressive position is to be worked through, and the object is to be allowed its independence. In unconscious phantasy this means that the individual has to face his inability to protect the object. His psychic reality includes the realization of the internal disaster created by his sadism and the awareness that his love and reparative wishes are insufficient to preserve his object, which must be allowed to die with the consequent desolation, despair, and guilt. Klein (1935) put it as follows:

> Here we see one of the situations which I described above, as being fundamental for 'the loss of the loved object'; the situation, namely, when the ego becomes fully identified with its good internalized objects, and at the same time becomes aware of its own incapacity to protect and preserve them against the internalized persecuting objects and the id. This anxiety is psychologically justified.

These processes involve intense conflict which we associate with the work of mourning and which gives rise to anxiety and mental pain.

The depressive position can thus also be seen to contain gradations within it, particularly in relation to the question of whether loss is feared and denied or whether it is acknowledged and mourning is worked through. I have used this distinction to divide the depressive position into a phase of *fear of loss of the object* and a phase of *experience of the loss of the object* as follows:

Fear of loss of the object ⟷ Experience of loss of the object

Mourning

Freud (1917) has described the process of mourning in beautiful detail, and emphasizes that in the work of mourning it is the reality of the loss which has so painfully to be faced. In the process every memory connected with the bereaved is gone over and reality testing applied to it until gradually the full force of the loss is appreciated.

'Reality-testing has shown that the loved object no longer exists, and it proceeds to demand that all libido shall be withdrawn from its attachments to that object' (Freud 1917: 245). And later,

> Each single one of the memories and situations of expectancy which demonstrate the libido's attachment to the lost object is met by the verdict of reality that the object no longer exists; and the ego, confronted as it were with the question whether it shall share this fate is persuaded by the sum of the narcissistic satisfactions it derives from being alive to sever its attachment to the object that has been abolished.
>
> (Freud 1917: 255)

If successful, this process leads to an acknowledgement of the loss and a consequent enrichment of the mourner. When we describe the mourning sequence in more detail it can be seen to involve two stages which correspond to the two subdivisions of the depressive position I have outlined above.

First, in the early phases of mourning the patient attempts to deny the loss by trying to possess and preserve the object, and one of the ways of doing this, as we have seen, is by identification with the object. Every interest is abandoned by the mourner except that connected with the lost person, and this total preoccupation is designed to deny the separation and to ensure that the fate of the subject and the object is inextricably linked. Because of the identification with the object the mourner believes that if the object dies then he must die with it, and conversely, if the mourner is to survive, then the reality of loss of the object has to be denied.

The situation often presents as a kind of paradox because the mourner has somehow to allow his object to go even though he is convinced that he himself will not survive the loss. The work of mourning involves facing this paradox and the despair associated with it. If it is successfully worked through, it leads to the achievement of separateness between the self and the object because it is through mourning that the projective identification is reversed and parts of the self previously ascribed to the object are returned to the ego (Steiner 1990a). In this way the object is viewed more realistically, no longer distorted by projections of the self, and the ego is enriched by re-acquiring the parts of the self which had previously been disowned.

Klein (1940) has described this process vividly in the patient she calls Mrs A, who lost her son and after his death began sorting out her letters, keeping his and throwing others away. Klein suggests that she was unconsciously trying to restore him and keep him safe, throwing out what she considered to be bad objects and bad feelings. At first she did not cry very much and tears did not bring the relief which they did later on. She felt numbed and closed up, and she also stopped dreaming as if she wanted to deny the reality of her actual loss and was afraid that her dreams would put her in touch with it.

Then she dreamed that she saw a mother and her son. The mother was wearing a black dress and she knew that her son had died or was going to die.

This dream put her in touch with the reality not only of her feelings of loss but of a host of other feelings which the associations to the dream provoked, including those of rivalry with her son who seemed to stand also for a brother, lost in childhood, and other primitive feelings which had to be worked through.

Later she had a second dream, in which she was flying with her son when he disappeared. She felt that this meant his death – that he was drowned. She felt as if she too were to be drowned – but then she made an effort and drew away from the danger back to life.

The associations showed that she had decided that she would not die with her son, but would survive. In the dream she could feel that it was good to be alive and bad to be dead, and this showed that she had accepted her loss. Sorrow and guilt were experienced but with less panic since she had lost the previous conviction of her own inevitable death.[1]

We can see that the capacity to acknowledge the reality of the loss, which leads to the differentiation of self from object, is the critical issue which determines whether mourning can proceed to a normal conclusion. This involves the task of relinquishing control over the object, and means that the earlier trend which was aimed at possession of the object and denying reality has to be reversed. In unconscious phantasy this means that the individual has to face his inability to protect the object. His psychic reality includes the realization of the internal disaster created by his sadism and the awareness that his love and his reparative wishes are insufficient to preserve his object, which must be allowed to die, with the consequent desolation, despair, and guilt. These processes involve intense mental pain and conflict, which is part of the function of mourning to resolve.

Patient C

I will briefly mention another patient who had a long and very stuck analysis dominated by the conviction that it was imperative for him to

---

1 This description is particularly poignant because Melanie Klein wrote this paper shortly after she lost her own son in a mountaineering accident, and it is clear that Mrs A of the paper was actually herself (Grosskurth 1986).

become a doctor. In fact, he was unable to get a place at medical school, and after various attempts to study dentistry had to be content with a post as a hospital administrator, which he hated. Session after session was devoted to the theme of his wasted life and the increasingly remote possibility that studies at night school might lead to a place at a medical school, perhaps if not in this country then overseas.

I was able repeatedly to link his need to be a doctor to his conviction that he contained a dying object in his inner world which he considered he had to cure and preserve and that he could not accept his inability to do so. He could not recognize that this task was impossible and quite beyond his power, and he could not get on with his life and let his object die. He had a terrible fear that he would not be able to cope when his parents came to die and also a great fear of his own ageing and death. Somehow he was convinced that if he could be a doctor it would also mean that he would be immune from illness.

When he was 14 his grandmother developed a terrible fatal illness in which she gradually and slowly became paralysed and died. My patient could not bear to see this go on and especially could not bear to watch the loving way his grandfather cared for his wife. When the doctor broke the news to the family he ran out of the house in a panic. I had heard different references to this tragic experience over the years, and one day I interpreted that his wish to be a doctor was an omnipotent wish to reverse this death, and that he believed that he could even now keep his grandmother alive and was doing so inside himself through the fantasy that as a doctor he would cure her. He was for a moment able to follow me and seemed touched, but a few minutes later explained that his wish to be a doctor had occurred not then but years earlier at the age of 5 after he had his tonsils out. He described his panic as the anaesthetic mask was applied, and I have no doubt that he was afraid that he was going to die. The wish to be a doctor was therefore connected with the wish to preserve his own life as well as that of his objects, and the two were so inextricably linked that he could not consider that he could survive if his object were to die. The task of mourning could not proceed and the idea of relinquishing the ambition of being a doctor was tantamount to giving up the wish to live.

This patient seemed stuck in the first phase of the depressive position, and the pathological organization of the personality predominantly functioned as a defence against loss. He had a conviction that being a doctor would not only preserve his objects from illness and death but would also protect him. Because of the concreteness of his identifications he could not envisage letting his object die and surviving himself. It was just this which Mrs A achieved in the course of her mourning and it transformed her situation, allowing her to move from the phase of *fear of loss* to that of *experience of loss*. My patient was unable to make this transformation and was consequently unable to work through his mourning and proceed to the second phase of the depressive position.

Patient D

In other patients, even early in our contact with them, evidence of the capacity to face the experience of loss becomes apparent. This seemed to be the case with a student who was referred for psychotherapy by a psychiatrist following an admission to hospital because of depression and suicidal ruminations. He gradually improved and returned to his home but was undecided if he should continue his studies. He came to the consultation obviously anxious and within a few seconds became extremely angry, perhaps because I had so far remained silent. When I asked him if he wanted to begin he grimaced and snapped, 'No!' At first I thought he looked quite psychotic since his lips were trembling with rage and he had great difficulty controlling himself. After a few minutes he got up and walked about the room looking at my books and pictures, and eventually stopped and picked up a picture of two men playing cards, and said, 'What game do you think these two are playing?' I interpreted that he felt he and I were playing a game and he wanted to know what was going on. He relaxed slightly and sat down again. He then said he felt I was adopting a technique which was imposed on me by the Tavistock Clinic and that I expected him to go along with it. I interpreted that he saw me as a kind of robot who mechanically did what I was told, and he agreed.

When I asked for a dream, he described one he had had when he was 15 and which remained extremely vivid. In the dream he was standing in a city which had been completely destroyed. Around him was rubble and twisted metal, but there were also small puddles of water and in these a rainbow was reflected in brilliant colours.

I interpreted that he felt a kind of triumph if he could destroy me and make out of me a robot, which meant to him that I was simply twisted metal with nothing human about me. He admitted that the mood in the dream was ecstatic, and I suggested that the triumph and exaltation were a way of denying the despair and destruction. He relaxed perceptibly and with additional work we could link the catastrophe in the dream to a time at the age of 15 when he returned home to be told that his parents were going to separate.

This patient was aware of his inability to preserve his objects so that his inner world was dominated by desolation and despair and peopled by damaged and destroyed objects which gave it the desolate appearance of a destroyed city. This filled him with such despair and guilt that he could not face it and the organization he deployed used manic and other defences to protect him from it. However, if these were contained in the interview he was able to make contact with his depression and with the analyst.

In this chapter I have developed the idea of a continuum between the paranoid-schizoid and the depressive positions to include subdivisions of each so that an equilibrium diagram can be constructed as follows:

Paranoid-schizoid position   ⟷   Depressive position

| Pathological fragmentation | ↔ | Normal splitting | ↔ | Fear of loss of the object | ↔ | Experience of loss of the object |

Each position can be thought to be in equilibrium with those on either side of it, and attempts can thus be made to follow movement between them. The equilibrium diagram can be expanded to include a psychic retreat as follows:

Psychic retreat

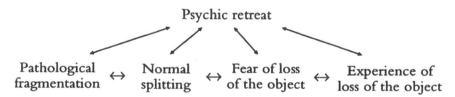

| Pathological fragmentation | ↔ | Normal splitting | ↔ | Fear of loss of the object | ↔ | Experience of loss of the object |

This type of diagram is meant as an aid to thinking about the patient and not as a tool for use during a session. Nevertheless, it is sometimes possible to observe movement in the mental organization of the patient, whether this is within a session or over weeks, months, or years of an analysis. He may emerge from a retreat only to return to its protection, but the anxieties he faces will also vary. In extremely disturbed patients most of the movement is between the retreat and states of pathological fragmentation. As development proceeds, other, less terrifying anxieties are faced, but the retreat may still be felt to be necessary if mental pain of an unbearable nature associated with fear of loss or the experience of loss has to be faced.

4

Review: narcissistic object relations and pathological organizations of the personality

In this chapter some of the previous work on psychic retreats and pathological organizations of the personality will be reviewed. The literature is so vast and the subject has been looked at from so many different points of view that I am not able to attempt a comprehensive survey, and I will, for the most part, restrict myself to those authors who have influenced me personally. The particular approach I have followed goes back to Freud's concern with the obstacles to progress in analysis most clearly expressed in 'Analysis terminable and interminable' (1937). Freud connected these obstacles with the operation of the death instinct, which he saw as setting an ultimate limit to the success of the individual's struggle with primitive destructive forces. These forces, which interfere with his capacity for love and creativity, threaten him from within and from without, and their reality may be so difficult to accept that omnipotent defences are mobilized to deal with them. It is these omnipotent defences struggling with primitive destructive elements in the personality which create the most serious problems in analysis and which become manifest in pathological organizations of the personality. The most important of these omnipotent defences later came to be studied under the heading of projective identification but was already implicit in the early studies of narcissism and narcissistic object relations. The work on narcissism again began with Freud (1910, 1914) but was developed by Abraham (1919, 1924) in his study of narcissistic resistance, and by Reich (1933) in his work on character analysis and his introduction of the idea of a 'character armour'. These studies led on to those of Melanie Klein and her successors, of whom Bion, Rosenfeld, Segal, and Joseph have been particularly influential.

It is important to recognize that this Kleinian approach is only one among many held by analysts who have studied the same and related areas of mental life. For example, obstacles to progress and to contact have often been studied under the heading of 'character disorder' and 'character resistance'. Sometimes different diagnostic types of character structure are examined, and an important contributor in this area is Kernberg (1967, 1975, 1976, 1979, 1983), who has described in detail distinct groups of narcissistic and borderline patients. To each of these he prescribed specific treatment strategies, some of which involve significant departures from classical psychoanalytic technique. Kernberg believes it is possible to define specific types of personality organization and to allocate patients accordingly. His work stresses different types of pathological organization of the personality, whereas mine attempts to identify features which are common to them all.

Many other writers have described character disorders from a variety of perspectives; for example, Nunberg (1956), Leowald (1962, 1978), Gitelson (1963), Loewenstein (1967), Giovacchini (1975, 1984), and Cooper (1986). Lax (1989) provides a review of some of this work which links obstacles to progress in analysis with character defences.

The study of developmental stages and the effect of fixations and regressions to these is another approach which is widely used to study the problem of stuck states and of patients being out of contact. Here the work of Balint (1968) and Winnicott (1958, 1965, 1971) brings an emphasis on regressions to states of mind in which development is slow or non-existent. Winnicott has, in addition, studied the situation where real contact with the patient is obstructed by the development of a 'false self' (Winnicott 1960), building on the description by Deutsch (1942) of the 'as–if' personality. Of particular importance in the study of psychic retreats is the work of Winnicott on transitional objects and transitional spaces (Winnicott 1953, 1971). There are many similarities between transitional spaces and psychic retreats but also some central differences. In particular is the value given by Winnicott to the transitional area which he sees as a place of cultural and personal development. In my approach, I emphasize them as areas of retreat from reality where no realistic development can take place. In my view, the retreat often serves as a resting place and provides relief from anxiety and pain but it is only as the patient emerges from the retreat that real progress can occur.

Many writers have made links with research in child development and this area of study has been greatly influenced by the work of Margaret Mahler (Mahler, Pine and Bergman 1975; Lax, Bach and Burland 1980). Her study of 'separation–individuation', which is concerned with separation anxiety and the development of a sense of separateness in infants and small children, is of particular relevance. A somewhat different approach which also relates developmental

41

pathologies with mental structures and organizations is that of Fonagy, who introduces the important concept of 'theory of mind' to discuss the child's development of the capacity to view his objects as real persons with mental states of their own. Fonagy (1991) discusses this idea in relation to the pathology of a borderline man who was traumatized as a child, and with Moran (Fonagy and Moran 1991) describes developmental processes which are responsible for various forms of failure to develop, leading to borderline pathology.

I decided that a thorough survey of these and many other related writings would take me too far from the central aim of this book, and I found that it was also not practical to review some of the basic concepts which have arisen out of the work of Klein and her followers. In particular, the reader is assumed to have some understanding of 'projective identification' (Klein 1946; Rosenfeld 1971b; Feldman 1992; Spillius 1988a and 1988b) and 'containment' (Bion 1959, 1962a; 1963; Britton 1992) which are essential to a full understanding of pathological organizations of the personality.

Narcissistic object relations and projective identification

One of the consequences of projective identification is that the subject relates to the object not as a separate person with his own characteristics but as if he is relating to himself. He may ignore aspects of the object which do not fit the projection or he may control and force or persuade the object to enact the role required of him. This type of narcissistic relationship was described by Freud (1910) in his study of Leonardo and elaborated in his paper on narcissism (1914). He showed how Leonardo treated his apprentices as if they represented *himself as a boy*. At the same time he identified with his mother and related to the boy as he wished his mother had related to him. Freud puts it as follows (1910):

> The child's love for his mother cannot continue to develop consciously any further; it succumbs to repression. The boy represses his love for his mother: he puts himself in her place, identifies himself with her, and takes his own person as a model in whose likeness he chooses the new objects of his love . . . boys whom he loves in the way in which his mother loved *him* when he was a child. He finds the objects of his love along the path of *narcissism* as we say; for Narcissus, according to the Greek legend, was a youth who preferred his own reflection to everything else and who was changed into the lovely flower of that name.
>
> (1910: 100)

A study of the narcissistic type of object relationship makes it clear that multiple identifications are involved. In the case of Leonardo an infantile part of the self is projected and identified with the apprentice, while remaining elements of the self are identified with the mother. In other cases, or in the same person at other times, the identifications can shift, and we often see the reversed picture – namely, that the maternal part of the self is projected and identified with an object while the self assumes an infantile identity. Joseph (1985) has drawn our attention to the need to consider what she calls 'the total situation' in these cases, and analysts often need to remind themselves that there is more than one way in which elements of the personality can become distributed among the objects with which the patient is in a relationship.

Narcissistic types of object relationship have been described by many writers. Abraham (1919) discusses narcissism as a prominent source of resistance in analysis, and after him Reich (1933) in his description of character armour stressed the defensive function of narcissistic relationships. Rosenfeld (1964, 1971a), who has emphasized the connection with projective identification, has shown how it can involve the idealization of good aspects but also of destructive parts of the self.

In his early paper on the psychopathology of narcissism Rosenfeld emphasizes defences against separateness and assumes that the mechanism by which separateness is denied is projective identification. He writes as follows:

> In narcissistic object relations defences against any recognition of separateness between self and object play a predominant part. Awareness of separation would lead to feelings of dependence on an object and therefore to anxiety. Dependence on an object implies love for, and recognition of, the value of the object, which leads to aggression, anxiety and pain because of the inevitable frustrations and their consequences. In addition dependence stimulates envy, when the goodness of the object is recognized. The omnipotent narcissistic object relations therefore obviate both the aggressive feelings caused by frustration and any awareness of envy. When the infant omnipotently possesses the mother's breast, the breast cannot frustrate him or arouse his envy. Envy is particularly unbearable to the infant and increases the difficulty in admitting dependence and frustration. . . .
>
> When the patient claims to possess the analysis, as the feeding breast, he gives himself credit for all the analyst's satisfactory interpretations, a situation which is experienced as perfect or ideal because it increases the patient's feeling during the analytic session that he is good and important. . . . All these patients seem to have in

common the feeling that they contain all the goodness which would otherwise be experienced in a relationship to an object.

(1964: 171–2)

We can see that projective identification gives rise to a state in which true separateness is not experienced. This state of mind provides relief from anxiety and from frustration as well as from envy, and is idealized. Often the patient believes that the analyst is also spared these unpleasant emotions and assumes that he too idealizes the narcissistic relationship.

Sometimes projective identification can be used in a more global way in which the whole self is felt to be projected into the object. Rosenfeld (1983) refers to this as a symbiotic type of object relationship in which the patient appears to live inside his object, sometimes accompanied by a phantasy that the analyst welcomes this kind of intrusion and reciprocates. More often the intrusion is a destructive one which is resented by the object, and the true nature of the relationship which results is a parasitic one. The patient may, however, idealize it and in this way the destructive nature of the projective identification is denied.

A type of narcissistic organization based on destructiveness was described by Meltzer (1968), who emphasized the cruelty and tyranny but had not yet appreciated the complexity of the organization involved. Discussing an addictive relationship to a bad part of the self which involves a submission to tyranny, he writes:

An illusion of safety is promulgated by the omniscience of the destructive part and perpetuated by the sense of omnipotence generated by the perversion or addictive activity involved. The tyrannical, addictive bad part is *dreaded*. It is important to note that, while the tyrant may behave in a way that has a resemblance to a persecutor, especially if any sign of rebellion is at hand, the essential hold over the submissive part of the self is by way of a dread of loss of protection against terror.

(1968: 105–6)

Later (Meltzer 1973), he describes the tyranny exerted by the narcissistic organization as follows:

The destructive part of the self then presents itself to suffering good parts first as a protector from pain, second as servant to its sensuality and vanity, and only covertly – in the face of resistance to regression – as the brute, the torturer.

(1973: 93)

It was, however, Rosenfeld (1971a) in his paper on destructive narcissism who gave the definitive description of this type of narcissistic object relationship based on idealization of destructive parts of the self. This important paper focuses on the problem of dealing with internal and external sources of destructiveness, which Rosenfeld relates to the activity of the death instinct. This theme goes back to Freud's early ideas on the death instinct which were elaborated by Melanie Klein. Although phrased in the now unfashionable language of instinct theory, the basic problem remains central to our understanding of the deepest roots of severe pathology. It postulates the universal emergence of internal sources of destructiveness manifested as primitive envy and threatening to destroy the individual from within. The part of the ego containing such impulses and phantasies is split off and evacuated by projective identification and in this way attributed to others. In the process, paranoid anxieties are created as the envious, destructive impulses are felt to attack the ego from without and a variety of defences are mounted in order to deal with this process.

Rosenfeld showed that it is not only good elements of the ego in relationship with good elements in the object which are idealized but that destructive elements can be similarly treated and that this con-stitutes a major way of dealing with destructiveness. He argues that a weak, dependent part of the self (the libidinal self) attempts to make contact with the analyst but is prevented from doing so by an alliance of destructive parts of the self in conjunction with destructive objects. This alliance he refers to as a narcissistic organization and he describes how it is often represented in the patient's material as an unconscious phantasy of a gang or Mafia which is idealized and which presents itself to the libidinal self as a helper or ally. In fact these destructive elements take over the personality and prevent any development and growth.

They may take a psychotic form and offer the patient a delusional world where freedom from pain and anxiety are promised, and their chief aim is often revealed as that of maintaining their hold on the personality and of preventing any real contact with the good analyst and constructive analytic work. Rosenfeld writes:

> This psychotic structure is like a delusional world or object, into which parts of the self tend to withdraw. It appears to be dominated by an omnipotent or omniscient extremely ruthless part of the self, which creates the notion that within the delusional object there is complete painlessness but also freedom to indulge in any sadistic activity. . . .

> The destructive impulses within this delusional world sometimes appear openly as overpoweringly cruel, threatening the rest of the self with death to assert their power, but more frequently they

appear disguised as omnipotently benevolent or life-saving, promising to provide the patient with quick ideal solutions to all his problems. These false promises are designed to make the normal self of the patient dependent on or addicted to his omnipotent self, and to lure the normal sane parts into this delusional structure in order to imprison them.

(Rosenfeld 1971a: 175)

This theme and the function of psychotic organizations are further discussed in Chapter 6.

Several authors have been influenced by Rosenfeld and have extended his findings. Thus Brenman (1985) has shown how a narcissistic organization leads to a narrowing of the perception of objects in which many aspects of their reality are not recognized. He was concerned with a patient in whom cruelty played an important role, and suggested that it was the goodness of the patient which was hijacked and perverted to the side of cruelty in order to give it strength and to avoid catastrophe.

Sohn (1985) emphasizes the way narcissistic organizations involve complex and relatively stable identifications via projective identification, in which the person feels that he becomes the object so that he believes, consciously or unconsciously, that he possesses all the goodness and other qualities of the object. This type of concretely possessed object exists within the patient and is a major source of omnipotence; Sohn refers to it as an 'identificate'. The relationship between the needy dependent parts of the self and the omnipotent narcissistic part is again seen as a perverse one. Sohn illustrates it by the apt image of the Pied Piper.

It is as if a Pied Piper process is at hand, with the dependent parts of the personality constantly being led away to disappearance, leaving the personality like the crippled boy who survived in the story. Simultaneously the same crippling is directed against the analytic work.

(1985: 205)

Rosenfeld recognized that these narcissistic states are responsible for much of the impasse in analysis which he studied in his later work. To some extent the views expressed in his final book (Rosenfeld 1987) changed to put more emphasis on trauma and especially on the way an early traumatic situation is repeated in the analysis by the actions of the analyst. In my view he went somewhat too far in this direction (Steiner 1989b), but his description of destructive narcissism is the basis of my formulation of pathological organizations of the personality. The elements I go on to emphasize are those which give this structure its highly organized state, and this aspect has also been described by a variety of writers. It is possible to see the existence of pathological organizations of the personality as a complex measure designed to deal with the problem of internal destructiveness, and the study of this subject was greatly advanced by Rosenfeld's work on destructive narcissism.

Pathological organizations of the personality

Perhaps it would be simpler to consider the whole literature on pathological organizations of the personality under the heading of 'narcissistic organizations', but a number of authors have stressed the organized nature of the defensive processes while describing essentially similar mental structures. They have tended to avoid the term 'narcissistic' and to prefer to stress the organized nature of the defences by speaking of 'defensive' or 'pathological' organizations. At the same time they have been aware that such complex structures depend on pathological splitting and projective identification, which implies that a narcissistic type of object relation is involved. Spillius (1988a) reprints several of the relevant papers in this area and provides a clear and insightful commentary on these issues. I will discuss a few of the major contributions in some detail to show some of the influences on my own ideas.

Riviere (1936) is perhaps the first of the authors who studied narcissistic object relations and emphasized the highly organized structure which results from the way objects and defence mechanisms are linked together. In an early study of refractory patients, she dealt chiefly with manic defences, which she saw as the result of narcissistic object relations similar to those described by Abraham (1919). Much of her paper deals with the way manic defences protect the patient from the despair and mental pain of the depressive position and she gives special emphasis to the organized nature of the defences.

> Observation has led me to conclude that where narcissistic resistances are very pronounced, resulting in the characteristic lack of insight and absence of therapeutic results under discussion, these resistances are in fact part of a *highly organized system of defence* against a more or less unconscious depressive condition in the patient and are operating as a mask and disguise to conceal the latter.
>
> (Riviere 1936: 138)

Here Riviere emphasizes the defence against depressive anxieties which confirms the well-established link between mania and depression. I will argue later that pathological organizations of the personality also protect the patient from the anxieties of the paranoid-schizoid position, and indeed may evolve primarily to deal with these more primitive states. This is clear in the cases described by Segal (1972) and O'Shaughnessy (1981).

Segal (1972) described a pathological organization of the personality based on omnipotence. The patient was not overtly psychotic, perhaps protected by obsessional elements which formed part of the organization, but the delusional system which served as a mad refuge was grossly psychotic and functioned as a defence against the re-emergence of a catastrophic situation. Although her patient was clearly extremely disturbed, many of the features of the organization she described are observable in less ill patients.

Segal's patient suffered from severe obsessional ceremonials, and was preoccupied with a mission – namely, to convert people to Christianity – for which task he had to be perfectly efficient. To this end he pursued a number of activities he called 'operations' which supported his idea that he was a great strategist. These were varied and numerous but all could be seen to be anti-analysis, and the analyst was seen as someone on the side of reality and hence a threat to his operations. All of these could be seen as attempts at creating an *'inside the womb'*, or sometimes *'inside the bottom'*, existence, where he had an exciting relationship with a 'magic father penis'. Coming out of this situation was fraught with disaster, and Segal linked this with a disastrous experience in infancy where an abrupt weaning was closely followed by the death of his father and the depression and subsequent absence of his mother. She considered that these events must have given rise to murderous and cannibalistic fantasies and a conviction that he had murdered both his parents, so that for him to get in touch with any human feelings of love or dependence was linked with the expectation of a catastrophic ending.

Perverse aspects dominated the transference of Segal's patient, in particular an extreme sadism which had many of the elements of the narcissistic gang described by Rosenfeld (1971a). He would, for instance, say to his analyst, 'Hitler knew how to deal with you people,' in a way that would make her experience a momentary flood of hatred. Moreover, the cruelty was associated with phantasied relationships with powerful, cruel figures with whom he would identify. For example, a paratrooper who boasted of machine-gunning civilians in Cyprus for fun became an object of intense admiration and desire, and with this kind of partner he engaged in homosexual and masochistic practices.

48

An infantile self became known to Segal and her patient as 'baby Georgie', but any experience with it of a positive transference was violently attacked. Thus the patient killed small animals if hurt to prevent them suffering, and this was seen as an attack on the infantile part of the self. Analysis became a struggle to rescue this infantile self from the delusional omnipotent organization. Awareness of dependence led to fear of catastrophic weaning, and when interpretation did give rise to insight it led to horrifying feelings of emptiness.

Much of his omnipotent activity was based on a need to restore lost objects and lost functions of the ego in a manner reminiscent of Freud's account of the Schreber case (1911a). Segal uses the term 'restitution' rather than 'reparation' because destructive elements dominated and the whole system was an attack on reality. It was therefore much more centred on the paranoid–schizoid position, and elements of love and concern for the object which predominate in depressive reparation here played a very minor role, although they were not entirely absent.

Finally, Segal points out a feature which is characteristic of most if not all pathological organizations of the personality, when she shows that, although introduced to avoid a catastrophe, it was the organization itself which became a chronic catastrophe.

> It is the existence of the system that prevented him from making contact with such aspects of his mother as were available to him and from renewing any real contact with her after her return. . . . Baby Georgie and his potential for growth were stunted not by the 'catastrophe' but by the delusional system developed to prevent the recurrence of the catastrophe.
>
> (Segal 1972: 400)

O'Shaughnessy (1981), discussing a less psychotic, but also for a time a very stuck patient, gives a detailed description of a defensive organization which functioned to protect her patient from contact and hence from anxiety. She stresses the way patients may seek an analysis because they need a refuge against contact with themselves and their objects. They then use the analysis to re-establish a defensive organization which serves as such a refuge against objects internal and external which are causing them nearly overwhelming anxiety.

Her patient went through four phases in his analysis. In the first phase the defensive organization had broken down and failed to provide the desired protection, giving rise to a desperate situation leading to confusion and overwhelming anxieties. He felt threatened and longed for stillness and unchangingness, and felt a need to regain his defensive organization.

In the second period, the organization was re-established in the analysis, leading to relief at the cost of restricted object relations. Like Riviere (1936), O'Shaughnessy emphasizes the way relief was achieved by the interlocking use of several defences, omnipotent control, and denial, and several forms of splitting and projective identification, to organize relations within himself and between himself and objects.

In the third phase, O'Shaughnessy observed an exploitation of the defensive organization for the gratification of cruelty and narcissism, resulting in states similar to those described by Segal (1972) and Rosenfeld (1971a).

Finally, during the eighth year of the analysis there were growing signs of a more alive, less restricted contact, and the emergence of some trusted objects enabled the patient to go forward in his development.

In this compelling paper O'Shaughnessy makes several points which are fundamental to the understanding of pathological organizations of the personality. First, she showed how in her patient the organization served to create a refuge which led to a longed-for state of relative tranquillity. When it broke down, confusion and anxiety dominated, and when it was re-established, she showed how it was used to perpetuate a perverse relationship with the analyst. Like Riviere and Segal, she stresses the highly organized nature of the defensive system and the desperate quality of the anxiety which threatens the individual if the organization breaks down.

She raises the question as to whether the organization actually helps the patient to develop by providing the longed-for sanctuary from anxiety and from contact, and suggests that perhaps, in the conditions provided by analysis, it was able to do this. A most significant point arises from her description of the fate of the organization when development did occur. This did not mean that the organization was dismantled; instead, a split in the personality developed and, despite the continued existence of the pathological organizations of the personality, a part of the patient which was able to stay in contact with his object and with reality was strengthened. An omnipotent part of the patient continued to prefer to stay in projective identification with powerful destructive objects and was obstructive and contemptuous of realistic efforts to develop. O'Shaughnessy considers that the existence of this type of split is a characteristic aftermath of a defensive organization. Her patient, when persecuted or over-guilty, tended abruptly to lose interest in his object and to become omnipotent and perverse, but such changes became more temporary and he was less under the sway of the organization.

In a later paper O'Shaughnessy (1993) uses the term 'enclave' to describe something very similar to a psychic retreat. She is particularly concerned with the way the patient persuades the analyst into a restricted part object relationship which is limited and over close. Such relationships may be idealized in a harmonious way which is difficult for the analyst to avoid. She contrasts such 'enclaves' with what she calls 'excursions', namely more or less successful attempts by the patient to induce the analyst to move away from areas of great anxiety to activity which avoids contact with anxiety. I believe enclaves and excursions are fundamentally similar and that both are varieties of psychic retreat and manifestations of a pathological organization of the personality.

Riesenberg-Malcolm (1981) discusses a particular type of mental organization in which perverse masochistic elements predominate. The patient turns to self-punishment in an attempt to use expiation and suffering to avoid a perception of the damaged state of his internal objects and in this way to evade guilt. This punishment takes the place of what instead should be reparation – that is, restoration of internal objects that have been attacked in phantasy; the self-punishment serves as a further attack on the object and as a result the guilt is increased and not lessened and leads to an impasse.

The theme of a powerful destructive part of the self which tyrannizes the dependent needy part of the self and prevents it from gaining access to good objects is central to most of the work in this area. The perverse nature of this relationship between elements in the self is mentioned by all the writers in this field and is the chief emphasis of Riesenberg-Malcolm. It is, however, Joseph (1982,1983) who has studied these perverse relationships in greatest detail and shows how patients' suffering can be used to triumph over that side of them capable of development and of a relationship to life and to the good objects which represent it. The way in which a pathological organization of the personality can serve as a refuge is well illustrated in a dream from her Patient A described in her paper entitled 'Addiction to near death'.

> He was in a long kind of cave almost a cavern. It was dark and smoky and it was as if he and other people had been taken captive by brigands. There was a feeling of confusion, as if they had been drinking. They, the captives, were lined up along a wall and he was sitting next to a young man. This man was subsequently described as looking gentle, in the mid-twenties, with a small moustache. The man suddenly turned towards him, and grabbed at him and at his genitals as if he were homosexual, and was about to knife my patient, who was completely terrified. He knew that if he tried to resist the man would knife him and there was tremendous pain.
>
> (Joseph 1982: 129–30)

The role of perversion in pathological organizations of the personality is of central importance, and in my view is one of the elements which holds the organization together. It will be further discussed in Chapters 8 and 9. Sometimes, as in O'Shaughnessy's patient, the refuge provided by the pathological organizations of the personality offers the seduction of peace and calm, but sometimes, as in Joseph's Patient A, the refuge is a terrifying one and nevertheless is turned to as if the patient is addicted to it. Partly this is because of the pull of the masochism providing a sexual gratification from being in such pain and from being dominated, but another critical factor is the way the pull towards life and sanity is got rid of by projection into the analyst.

The structure of the organization is based on splits in the personality which result in parts of the self being in identification with objects and in alliances with objects in complex ways. Thus Joseph describes how her patient was dominated by an aggressive part of himself that not only attempted to control and destroy her work but that was actively sadistic towards other parts of the self which would be more available for help were they not masochistically caught up in the perversion.

Rey (1975, 1979) has made a particular study of schizoid states and schizoid modes of being, which are closely related to pathological organizations of the personality. He uses the word 'schizoid', in the tradition of Fairbairn (1949) and Guntrip (1968), to emphasize states of mind in which splitting predominates and also to refer to a particular type of borderline patient who tends to be out of contact with himself and his objects (Steiner 1979).

The term 'borderline' in Rey's work refers not only to a category of patients but to a particular aspect of the mental structure of these patients and to the location of the self in that structure. He describes how his patients feel themselves to be neither fully inside nor fully outside their objects. They exist in a borderline area which corresponds to what I have called a psychic retreat. In this area they are protected from anxiety but have grave problems of identity so that they feel neither fully sane nor quite mad, neither completely male nor quite female, neither homosexual nor heterosexual, neither children nor adults, neither small nor big, neither loving nor hating, but existing on the border between these conditions. Rey summarizes this by stating:

> It seems that those people represent a group of persons who have achieved a kind of stability of personality organization in which they live a most limited and abnormal emotional life which is neither neurotic nor psychotic but a sort of frontier state.
>
> (Rey 1979: 450)

Rey (1975) has made an important contribution to the understanding of psychic retreats by describing the way mental space is structured. He suggests that the infant at birth continues to live in a space surrounded by his mother's care, which, by analogy with the kangaroo's pouch, he calls the 'marsupial space', and a full psychological birth does not take place until the infant differentiates for himself a personal space as a separate entity from the maternal space. The borderline patient often feels he has been prematurely and cruelly pushed out of this maternal space and attempts to regain his right to reside there. This may emerge as a demand to have access to the analyst's circle of friends, to his house or his bed, but, because of the extremely concrete thinking these patients are forced to use, the underlying phantasy may be to live in a cavity of the analyst's body. Access to these spaces may be felt as dependent on the analyst's good will, and the patient may have assiduously avoided any behaviour that would make him fear he is no longer allowed in this favoured position. Separation is then experienced as a terrible expulsion, since this interior is idealized as a wonderful dream place where the analyst does the worrying, and expulsion is felt as being pushed out prematurely to starvation, cold, and death. These thoughts are clearly of great relevance to the origin of psychic retreats and their relationship, at a primitive level, to phantasies about the mother's body.

Alternately, when these patients feel they have seduced, cajoled, or deceived the analyst into colluding with their demand to live in what is felt to be his space, they begin to feel afraid of the closeness. They feel that their minds have been taken over, that they have got into a mad state, that they have lost their freedom, that their need makes them a prisoner of a crazy kind of analysis, so that they feel trapped and unable to escape. Rey describes this situation and calls it the 'claustro-agoraphobic' dilemma (Rey 1975; Steiner 1979). He recognizes, in this way, that the refuge can appear as a place of safety when the patient is outside it and at the same time become a persecuting place where he feels trapped when he is inside it. Sometimes the claustro-agoraphobic dilemma makes the patient feel that they can find no place where they feel truly secure. In some patients this dilemma is observable as a rapid oscillation between a claustrophobic and an agoraphobic existence. While trapped in a psychic retreat they feel claustrophobic, but as soon as they manage to escape they once again panic and return to their previous position.

5

The recovery of parts of the self lost through projective identification: the role of mourning[1]

In previous chapters I have described how the function of a retreat – namely, to prevent contact with pain and anxiety – is related to its structure and how this structure in turn depends on a complex set of interlocking object relationships which become internalized as a permanent feature of the individual's personality. The stability and rigidity of such structures arise from the fact that projective identification is used in ways which make it more or less irreversible. Parts of the self are split off and projected into objects where they permanently reside, remaining unavailable to the self. Objects containing these elements of the self have a particular concreteness (Segal 1957) and make up the building blocks from which the retreat is constructed. In particular, they are welded together into a narcissistic group and form a pathological organization of the personality. In the process, the ego is weakened through the unavailability of these split-off elements and becomes even more dependent on the organization by virtue of this weakness.

The result of projective identification used in this way is markedly different from the normal situation where it is deployed flexibly and reversibly. In this chapter I will present some clinical material to illustrate the way parts of the personality can become almost totally unavailable through this process. After this, I will discuss some of the factors which make the organization so stable and which prevent the reversibility of projective identification and consequently obstruct the return of lost parts of the self. This will involve a detailed discussion of the process of mourning which, in my view, plays an essential role in the recovery of parts of the self lost in this way. If the patient *is* able to

---

1 Parts of this chapter are based on material previously published in a paper entitled 'The aims of psychoanalysis' (Steiner 1989a).

deal with loss by mourning he can, in the process, regain lost parts of the self, while if he is unable to mourn, the projective identification remains irreversible and the lost part of the self remains embedded in the object into which it has been projected. I will argue that those factors which obstruct mourning at the same time obstruct the return of projected elements.

Clinical material

Mrs B was a middle-aged woman who filled her sessions with complaints and resentments, and produced an atmosphere of emptiness and despair by adopting a kind of thoughtless, whining attitude and manner of speaking which made me feel it was impossible for her to think intelligently. For example, she would moan, 'Why don't you tell me what to do?'; and having read in a book on psychoanalysis that patients were supposed to free associate she complained, 'You didn't tell me I should free associate. I have been coming all these years and I never knew what I was supposed to do.'

She was chronically unhappy, and many of her sessions were filled with detailed descriptions of a variety of somatic complaints and long accounts of her misfortunes. The resentments mostly had to do with her childlessness and her relative poverty, and involved the painful comparison with her ex-husband who had gone on to remarry and have children and whose successful business she read about periodically in the newspaper.

In fact, similar resentments had been present all her life and she felt her older sister was favoured. Except on holidays the parents had separate rooms and she had shared her mother's bed until she was given her own room when she was 8 years old. Much of the resentment seemed to date from this time, when she became more aware of her rivalry with her sister and her father, and seemed never to have really felt loved again.

Her father was a headmaster who was also the leader of a small, obscure, but very powerful religious sect, and he created an atmosphere of severity and sobriety in which sin had to be searched for everywhere and stamped out and resisted. At home it was impossible to rebel against this climate, but the patient did well at school and, unlike her sister, went on to university where in her first year she surprised everyone with her talent in science. This independence reflected a capacity to think for herself and appeared to threaten her equilibrium, to the extent that at the beginning of her second year she had a breakdown and was sent home in an acute anxiety state with depersonalization and some persecutory thoughts. She gradually improved but could not return to college and after two years off began a secretarial course as her sister had done.

It was difficult to believe that the whining, helpless, miserable woman I listened to in the analytic sessions could have excelled in science at the university, and it was only as I got glimpses of a quite superior intelligence – for example, when she mastered complex and subtle problems at work, or when she was able to correct me on a logical point in an interpretation – that I began to realize that she had done something with her capacity to think. In part, she seemed to split it off and project it into me so that she came to depend on me for the most elementary thought; one of the factors behind this projection seemed to be the conviction that thinking was dangerous. It is clear that she had not in any way destroyed her intelligence because, when she caught me out doing something wrong, she would pounce with a clear and incisive thrust to show me how wrong I had been, but for everyday purposes and particularly in the analytic work her capacity to think was unavailable to her. Thinking was permitted if it did not challenge an existing order which preserved her status quo, but she could not think for herself and she had to make it clear that it was unfair to expect her even to attempt this.

One day she arrived five minutes late explaining that she had been struggling to get away from a friend who wanted to talk and this had delayed her.

She then described a dream in which she was descending to the underground and at the foot of the steps found herself having to make a choice between the left-hand passage leading to town and the right-hand one leading home. She stood there, in the dream, unable to choose, feeling terribly heavy, and found that she had a gardening sickle in her hand. Her indecision made her late and she was relieved, since this meant she did not have time to go to town and could go home and do the work she needed to do in the garden which was terribly overgrown and untidy.

The sickle had been lent to her by a neighbour some two years previously and she discovered it a few days before while clearing out her garden shed. She felt guilty not only that she had not returned it but that she had never used it. She described it as a horrible sharp thing and wondered why the neighbour had not asked for it back.

I interpreted that the choice in the underground in her dream represented the conflict she was in between doing the painful analytic work and fleeing from it, and the heaviness she felt seems to have been connected with the strain of the conflict. I connected her lateness, due to the difficulty in tearing herself away from her friend, with her reluctance to leave a comfortable situation and use her intelligence in the session where, as in her garden at home, there was a lot of work to be done. Her response was to launch into a further outburst of whining and complaint. She ignored the essence of what I said and concentrated on the fact that I had mentioned that there was a lot of work still to be done in the analysis. She said that she felt heavy now and complained that my interpretations were not clear and persecuted her since, if a lot of work remained unfinished, she must still be very ill.

I suggested that part of her despair at the idea of work was connected with her fear of using her intelligence which she knew could be sharp and hurtful like the gardening sickle but was also necessary for useful work. I thought she was afraid to use her intelligence because she was afraid that it could be used to attack me more openly and that this would be dangerous. She preferred to leave the responsibility for thinking in me and to watch how I worked, pouncing on me when I did something wrong. She responded indignantly, at first, suggesting that it was a terrible thing to imply that a patient might attack her analyst, but her attempt to make me feel I had said something improper was unconvincing. It was reminiscent of the romantic atmosphere which dominated the early years of her treatment in which the inter-action was highly eroticised and then treated as something improper.

I thought that she was also afraid to think scientifically and to reach conclusions on the basis of evidence. If she did, she would have to evaluate what sort of analyst I was, and she was afraid that she would feel let down by what she found. This would inevitably be a dis-appointment in comparison with the romantic image she created of me. No doubt she would also ultimately have to come to terms with what *she* was like as well as what sort of man her husband was and what sort of parents and family she had. To recognize both positive and negative aspects of her objects she would have to clear away much confusion which was usually dealt with by romantic idealization, and which, I thought, was represented by the overgrowth in her garden.

A great deal of the interaction in the transference was dominated by this romantic, dreamy state in which everything was eroticized in a way that was both child-like and sadistic. When she behaved in this in-nocent, childish way she would secretly remain on guard and carefully looked after her own interests. Her constant complaints about her loneliness and her poverty seemed connected with the idea of a world of comfort and luxury which had been promised and then stolen from her. Much of this went back to the time when she shared her mother's bed and shared what she saw as a pampered life without the intrusion of a sexual father.

These attitudes were markedly present in the transference, and she would hint and occasionally admit that I had been incorporated into her romantic fantasies. Mostly, however, she would only complain that I could not really be interested in her because she was too old, or that I preferred professionally successful women. It was impossible to discuss these fantasies, and if I tried to do so she became indignant and accused me of having improper thoughts and of exploiting her trust and her innocence. It seemed to me that in this dream state she felt close to me in a vaguely eroticized way but that if this was mentioned the spell was broken and she felt expelled from the intimacy as she had been from her mother's bed.

She was able to use her intelligence if it complied with the organization's wishes; namely, to protect herself from any real contact and thus to preserve the status quo. Thinking for herself, having desires and taking responsibility for herself were forbidden and the capacity to carry out these activities was projected. In order to take back into herself these capacities she would have had to risk a rebellion against the organization, and I think this was what she attempted to do when she enjoyed the freedom of her first year at university. This rebellion ended in disaster, and subsequently thinking of an independent kind in her everyday life or in her analysis was seen as dangerous. My wish to work with her, and in particular my idea that she might accept responsibility for her own wishes and thoughts, were felt as a cruel attack and an indication of my unwillingness to carry out these functions for her. I was at these times treated as the representative of the rebellious wish to think for herself and had to be stopped. At other times I was provoked to act as part of a persecuting organization and she experienced me as demanding an unthinking obedience and agreement.

With repeated analysis of this kind of situation she did gradually come to acknowledge some of her own talents and capabilities, but progress was always elusive and left her feeling guilty and unprotected. To allow her thinking to be used incisively, like a sickle, was to allow a more real interaction which was experienced as a dangerous kind of intercourse. Intelligence, the capacity to observe, to make judgements, and to retain contact with reality seemed, in my patient, to lead her to recognize the state of her objects, and to recognize her own impulses, and this appeared to make her afraid of what she would feel and what she would do. She could protect herself by splitting off and projecting these capacities but in the process was seriously disabled.

When I was able to recognize that she was not stupid but had a high degree of competence which she was unable to use, it made me more hopeful that she could be helped and it was therefore a disappointment to find that she resisted this process with all the means she could find and that indeed a peculiar kind of perverse intelligence lay behind her pseudo-stupidity. This resistance seemed to be directed against the psychic reality which her intelligence led her to appreciate, as if she knew that facing this reality would ultimately put her in touch with life-and-death issues which she preferred to avoid or at least postpone. When she did use her intelligence in the service of the analytic work she had to face an internal and external situation which was barren and terrifying in its emptiness. She could then bring up memories of lost good experiences including her feelings at the actual death of her parents, but it also seemed to involve letting go of a state of mind in which she could retain control of her objects and live in a dream world with them. It seemed to me that the chief purpose of the projective identification I have described was to hold onto a relationship with me in which the intelligence and desire were mine, and her preoccupation was to ensure that, having been given this power, I was prevented from exploiting her either sexually or financially. To own her own impulses was equivalent to letting me go, which she felt she could not survive.

Discussion

Experience with this patient and others (for example, Mr C in Chapter 6) led me to connect the failure to take back parts of the self lost through projective identification, with a failure to relinquish an omnipotent control over the object. I linked this with Rosenfeld's (1964) emphasis on the narcissistic relationship as a defence against separateness, and it seemed to me that this process of relinquishment involved precisely the same stages as those which are involved in the mourning following a bereavement and which have been extensively studied since Freud's original exploration of them in 'Mourning and melancholia' (Freud 1917; Bowlby 1980; Parkes 1972). This led me to formulate the specific notion that in order to regain parts of the self lost through projective identification it is necessary to relinquish the object and mourn it. It is in the process of mourning that projective identification is reversed and the ego is enriched and integrated.

The re-acquisition of projected parts of the self

Bion's theory of the containing function of the object (Bion 1959, 1962a, 1963) allows us to recognize how, if the analyst is open to receive and contain the projected fragments, a relief of anxiety results. In this process the object can function to collect and integrate the disparate elements of the self as they are assembled after having been

59

projected into him. According to Bion's model (1962a), it is the analyst's capacity to understand and give meaning to the projected fragments which provides the containment and which transforms them into a tolerable form which the infant can then re-introject.

In the clinical material I have discussed it is possible to observe how this degree of understanding was, at least sometimes, achieved in the transference and that I found periodically that Mrs B did feel understood and as a result her anxiety was relieved. Moreover, she was able to work better and had a more integrated feel about her as the various functions she got rid of by projection were collected in the transference. She could internalize me as the container of the various functions she projected, but she could not relinquish hold of me or allow a true separateness to develop.

If the analyst can function as such a container, and register and give meaning to the projected fragments, an integration takes place and the patient feels less anxious and less fragmented as he feels understood. In this phase, however, the patient is dependent on the availability of the analyst to act as the container and to bring the parts together through giving them meaning. Bion (1962a) suggested that it is through being understood in this way that the patient can take the projections back into himself but I believe the patient continues to need the object to act as a container and that the projections are not truly withdrawn until a second stage is reached. What is internalized in the first stage is an object containing parts of the self so that true separateness is not yet achieved and the lessening of anxiety which results during this first stage depends on a narcissistic type of object relationship. Sometimes this situation results in the phenomenon of the 'eternal patient' who improves but only as long as he is 'in analysis'.

Such a division of the process of achieving separateness into two stages is related to the way the depressive position can be considered to have two stages. I described this in Chapter 3 and called these the stage where *fear* of the loss of the object is paramount and the stage where the *experience* of the loss of the object is worked through. The stage of containment corresponds to the first phase of the depressive position, where relief depends on the continuing presence of the object, and this is also apparent in the early stages of mourning following an actual bereavement and has to be successfully worked through for the second stage to be achieved. Studies of bereavement have outlined various stages in the process, but all agree that in the early stages attempts are made to deny the experience of loss and that this has to be overcome as the reality of the loss is faced (Bowlby 1980; Parkes 1972; Lindemann 1944). It is in the second stage, which represents a move towards independence, that the object has to be relinquished, and I believe that it is at this point that the projections are withdrawn from the object and returned to the self. This stage involves facing the loss of the object and consequently means that mourning must be worked through.

Mourning

In Chapter 3 I briefly discussed the sequence of events in mourning using Freud's description from 'Mourning and melancholia'. He describes how, following a bereavement, the loss of an object leads at first to an identification with the object and a denial of the loss, and he goes on to emphasize the importance of facing reality if mourning is to be worked through. In mourning it is the reality of loss which is so difficult to face, and Freud conceives of this in terms of libido, explaining that it is the libido's attachment to the lost object which is met by the verdict of reality.

Today, as we recognize the central role of projective identification in the creation of pathological object relations, we can review Freud's formulation while thinking more in terms of detachments of parts of the self from the object rather than in terms of detachment of libido. It then becomes clear that, as reality is applied to each of the memories of the lost object, what has to be faced is the painful recognition of what belongs to the object and what belongs to the self. It is through the detailed work of mourning that these differentiations are made, and in the process the lost object is seen more realistically and the previously disowned parts of the self are gradually acknowledged as belonging to the self.

If mourning can be worked through, the individual becomes more clearly aware of a separateness of self and object and recognizes more clearly what belongs to the self and what belongs to the object. When such separateness is achieved it has immense consequences, because along with it go other aspects of mental function which we associate with the depressive position, including the development of thinking and symbol formation (Bion 1962a; Segal 1957).

We can see that the capacity to acknowledge the reality of the loss, which leads to the differentiation of self from object, is the critical issue which determines whether mourning can proceed to a normal conclusion. This involves the task of relinquishing control over the object and means that the earlier trend, which was aimed at possession of the object and denying reality, has to be reversed. In unconscious phantasy this means that the individual has to face his inability to protect the object. His psychic reality includes the realization of the internal disaster created by his sadism and the awareness that his love and his reparative wishes are insufficient to preserve his object, which must be allowed to die with the consequent desolation, despair, and guilt. These processes involve intense mental pain and conflict, which are part of the function of mourning to resolve.

It is clear that what applies for the mourning connected with an actual bereavement is in its essentials also true for all experience of separateness which at a primitive level is felt as a loss. Thus when an infant faces rejections, disappointments, or separations from his mother, the infant believes he has lost her and, because of the omnipotence of his thoughts, has the phantasy that it is his murderous impulses which have killed her. If he is able to face the psychic reality of this loss and suffer the pain of mourning he can, in the process, withdraw projections back into himself. He is thereby strengthened and the object is internalized in a form less distorted by projective identification. In Chapter 3 I described a patient (Patient C) who could not face the death of his objects because it was so compounded with fears about his own death, and this can be a major issue in some patients. By contrast, Segal (1958) has described how the analysis of an old man's fear of death enabled him to work through some of his fears of the loss of his objects.

In analysis it is often breaks in continuity such as those which occur when the analyst is ill, or over weekends and holidays, which enable these processes to be studied, but the same things happen whenever the analyst is experienced as independent and separate, thinking for himself, and the patient has to face the reality of relinquishing possessive control over the analyst. It is often the capacity to have an independent thought which most represents the independence of the analyst. If this separateness can be achieved, a quantum of mourning takes place and a quantum of self is returned to the ego. If the ego is strengthened a benign cycle can then be established and a more flexible and a more reversible form of projective identification deployed.

Obstacles to the recovery of projected parts of the self

Many studies of bereavement discuss various factors which interfere with normal mourning, and these may affect either of the two stages I have put forward. Problems of containment arise if acting out on the part of the analyst becomes too disruptive so that anxiety and excitement replaces understanding and integration. They also arise if the analyst is not sufficiently sensitive to the patient's projections and blocks his mind to them or if he is made so anxious by them that he projects them back at the patient.

However, most of the problems occur as the second stage of mourning is faced, and it is the relinquishment of the object which provokes such resistance. My experience with Mrs B and with several other patients has led me to believe that, provided the analyst is well trained and avoids gross acting out, containment is at least partly achieved and that many of the obstacles to progress arise as the patient and analyst approach the second phase. The situation we see then is the familiar one of the stuck patient who is relatively free of anxiety, who often manages much better in his everyday life, but who becomes attached in a dependent, but denied, way to the analysis.

One of the factors which makes it so difficult for the patient to pass from the stage of containment to that of relinquishment arises from the fact that he has to let go of an object upon whom he continues to believe his survival depends. At this primitive level separation is indistinguishable from death, and if the object is to die and if it contains too much of the self which has been split off and projected into it, then the patient is afraid of losing *himself* in the process. He may then panic and cling onto the object and deny the loss, as if he can in that way prevent his own death. The situation seems to him to be unfair because he cannot take back the projections unless he can mourn, and he cannot let the object die and mourn it without taking back the projections (Steiner 1990a).

It is often difficult to help the patient work through this impasse but an understanding of the paradox is sometimes helpful. Often it is only if the analyst can relinquish his need for the patient to conform to his wishes and to think the situation through in a fresh way that the patient is encouraged also to attempt to think for himself. An understanding of the complex structure of pathological organizations of the personality may also enable the analyst to recognize some of the difficulties which the patient faces.

My patient clearly found reality very difficult to bear and, instead of facing it and allowing herself to develop, she idealized earlier periods of her life when she phantasied that she could control and possess her objects so that they could not frustrate her or leave her. She could not accept their loss and not only longed to regain the previous state but was bitterly resentful when the reality of her situation confronted her. She could never mourn her objects and let them go. Her resistance to this process was connected with a fear and a hatred of reality and took the form of denial and misrepresentation of reality. If reality cannot be faced, mourning cannot proceed and the patient cannot regain the parts of the self she has disowned.

6

The retreat to a delusional world: psychotic organizations of the personality[1]

Psychotic organizations reflect the extreme nature of the experiences which the psychotic patient has to contend with. They are characterized by intense anxiety which demands drastic measures so that omnipotent forces are mounted to create a retreat organized in a psychotic way in defiance of reality. Psychotic organizations are rarely completely successful or stable, and the anxieties which threaten the individual as the organization begins to break down are usually conspicuous. The catastrophic nature of such anxiety underlies the desperate dependence on the organization, the loss of which implies the return of uncontrolled panic associated with experiences of fragmentation and disintegration of the patient's self and his world.

Such extreme states arise when ordinary defensive measures fail, and this may happen under the pressure of either internal or external factors. The psychotic nature of the experience is underlined by the fact that destructive attacks are mounted on the mind itself, with the result that a fundamental disturbance in the relationship between the self and the external world is created. Freud himself (1911a, 1924) considered that psychosis followed from an internal catastrophe which resulted in the appearance of a *rent* in the relationship between the ego and reality. In keeping with this view, Bion (1957, 1962a) suggests that the psychotic, in his attempt to free himself from the experience of a hated and feared reality, attacks the perceiving ego; that is, that part of his mind concerned with the perception of reality. He goes on to

---

1 This chapter is based on a paper presented for a panel discussion at the International Congress of Psychoanalysis, Rome, 1989, and published subsequently (Steiner 1991). I owe the clinical material to a colleague from Europe, who discussed the case with me and who kindly gave me permission to use it.

describe how the attack leads to a fragmentation of both ego and objects. Particles of object, each containing projected elements of the ego, make up what Bion calls 'bizarre objects', which create a diffusely persecuting and terrifying atmosphere, akin to 'nameless dread'.

The need for relief from such a state is urgent, and the sense of anxiety and confusion is so powerful that a psychotic organization based on omnipotent delusional forces may be the only way to create order and give relief from the diffuse anxiety. The patient may recognize the retreat so created as mad but may nevertheless feel that it is better than the catastrophic anxiety he experiences outside it. In other cases the patient idealizes the delusional world and represents it as a desirable place in order to have it accepted as a retreat from the psychotic ordeals of disintegration and annihilation. True integration and security are felt to be impossible and, despite its delusional foundation, the retreat offers a measure of stability as long as the psychotic organization is not challenged.

It has long been recognized that many of the long-term features of a delusional psychosis are restorative and arise in the wake of an internal disaster. For example, both Freud and Bion emphasize that many of the symptoms of psychosis arise from attempts on the part of the patient to restore his damaged ego and to reconstitute a world which has been destroyed. Thus in the Schreber case Freud states that

> The end of the world is the projection of this internal catastrophe; his subjective world has come to an end since his withdrawal of his love from it. . . . And the paranoiac builds it again, not more splendid, it is true, but at least so that he can once more live in it. He builds it up by the work of his delusions. *The delusional formation which we take to be the pathological product, is in reality an attempt at recovery, a process of reconstruction.*
>
> (Freud 1911a: 70)

Later he was more specific, and stated that 'a fair number of analyses have taught us that *the delusion is found like a patch over the place where originally a rent had appeared in the ego's relation to the external world*' (Freud 1924: 151).

Bion also emphasizes that the psychotic patient seeks to restore his damaged world and that he feels impelled to hold onto objects containing parts of the self and bring them back in an attempt at restitution of the ego. Following the description of the creation of bizarre objects by projective identification, he states:

If he wishes to bring back any of these objects *in an attempt at restitution of the ego*, and in analysis he feels impelled to make the attempt, he has to bring them back by projective identification in reverse and by the route by which they were expelled.

(Bion 1957: 51)

These attempts to restore the ego are based on an omnipotent delusional restoration of the damage done to both ego and objects. Most commonly, a complex delusional system is created which relieves anxiety by the imposition of an arbitrary and often cruel order on the previously chaotic state. It sometimes appears as if the patient believes that the 'rent' between the ego and reality results from an attack on his mind, leaving a tear through which mental contents will fall out, leaving nothing more than an empty shell. The psychotic organization is then called in to repair the rent by providing a patch which makes the patient feel more whole and less in danger of disintegrating.

Although paranoid delusions may themselves be frightening, it is often remarkable that a patient in a vague and ill-defined persecutory mood with terrible anxiety and depersonalization may actually become quite calm when his anxieties have been organized into a delusional system. What appeared as a nameless and vague dread becomes converted into a clear-cut delusion of persecution with apparent relief (Berner 1991; Sims 1988).

The psychotic organization protects the patient from the terrors of psychotic fragmentation, and for a while may lead to an equilibrium in which the patient can cope, albeit at the cost of grave disability. However, such an equilibrium is almost never stable and the patient is always threatened with a breakdown of the psychotic organization and a return of the unbearable anxiety. Indeed, it is often when such an equilibrium breaks down that the patient seeks treatment which he hopes will re-establish the psychotic organization and, in order to do this, may draw the analyst into a collaboration with psychotic forces.

Although the detailed structure of psychotic organizations varies, its essential nature is similar to that described for pathological organizations in general. Fragments of self and of internal objects are projected into objects which are, in turn, assembled into a powerful organization. Because of the extent of the fragmentation, the intensity of the violence, and the power of the destructiveness and hatred, the organization is forced to rely in a crude way on omnipotent mechanisms. Thus sane parts of the personality are overwhelmed and forcibly recruited to participate in the psychosis.

The coexistence of the psychotic and non-psychotic personalities

Both Freud and Bion describe the coexistence of psychotic and non-psychotic parts of the personality in the psychotic patient, and both speak as if a sane and a psychotic person exist within the one individual.
  Thus Freud writes:

> The problem of psychosis would be simple and perspicuous if the ego's detachment from reality could be carried through completely. But this seems to happen only rarely, or perhaps never. Even in a state so far removed from the reality of the external world as one of hallucinatory confusion, one learns from patients after their recovery that at the time in some corner of their mind (as they put it), there was a sane person hidden, who, like a detached spectator, watched the hub–hub of illness go past him.
>
> (Freud 1940: 201)

The relationship between the two parts of the personality is complex and their aims are usually antagonistic. The psychotic part attempts to retain omnipotent control over the object in order to repair the ego, while the neurotic part attempts to face psychic reality and let go of the object. Bion puts it as follows:

> The non-psychotic personality was concerned with a neurotic problem, that is to say a problem that centred on the resolution of a conflict of ideas and emotions to which the operation of the ego had given rise. But the psychotic personality was concerned with the problem of repair of the ego.
>
> (Bion 1957: 56)

The non-psychotic person is capable of facing reality, in particular the reality of loss, and as a result is able to work through mourning and thus allow projected parts of the self to be returned to the ego. This means that a 'balanced introjection and projection' can take place, and by this I think Bion means that projective identification is used flexibly with constant movement consisting of projection into objects followed by a recovery of the self through a return of the fragments previously got rid of. Bion argues that this type of reversible projective identification is necessary for the development of the capacity for thinking.
  Even when rudimentary, such thinking takes account of objects, and, with its help, the non-psychotic personality enhances its capacity to tolerate reality and in this way to modify rather than to evade it (Bion 1962a). The individual can use the capacity to think to proceed further in the task of working through the mental pain, grief, guilt, and

67

other emotions which make up the depressive position (Klein 1952). Eventually he can conceptualize his objects as whole people with minds capable of a private experience, and this enables a humanity and compassion for others to develop (Fonagy 1991). Unlike the psychotic patient, he has the advantage of his capacity for symbolic function which makes true reparation possible. This is something denied to the psychotic patient, who can only envisage concrete restitution by means of omnipotent mechanisms (Segal 1957; Rey 1986).

The non-psychotic personality is not therefore obliged to resort to such damaging defences in his struggle with reality, although he does, of course, deploy defences, including projective identification. In the case of the neurotic, however, destructive attacks are less directed at his own mind, and the projected fragments do not remain imprisoned in objects, so that a more fluid type of alternation between projective and introjective processes occurs which involves repeated cycles of possession followed by relinquishment and loss.

One of the major threats to the hegemony of the psychotic organization comes from the patient's own sanity, and this is often projected and comes to be represented by the analyst and his work. As a result, the organization attempts to prevent such sanity gaining any support which might enable it to disturb the status quo. The patient often believes that the threat of psychotic disintegration is so great that the organization must not be challenged and in that case any emergence of sanity must be ruthlessly suppressed. However, at other times a more complex relationship between sane and psychotic elements in the personality arises. The patient's sanity and his respect for the analytic work may survive the psychotic attacks and become sufficiently strong that they cannot simply be overwhelmed by brute force. It is then that perverse mechanisms are likely to become operative and the sane parts of the patient have to be seduced, threatened, and invited to collude with the psychotic organization.

Rosenfeld (1971a) has described the way in which the sane part of the patient is drawn into the psychotic organization in the following terms; his description also illustrates the way the organization comes to serve as a retreat into which the patient can withdraw.

> This psychotic structure is like a delusional world or object, into which parts of the self tend to withdraw. It appears to be dominated by an omnipotent or omniscient extremely ruthless part of the self, which creates the notion that within the delusional object there is complete painlessness but also freedom to indulge in any sadistic activity. . . .
> The destructive impulses within this delusional world sometimes

68

appear openly as overpoweringly cruel, threatening the rest of the self with death to assert their power, but more frequently they appear disguised as omnipotently benevolent or life-saving, promising to provide the patient with quick ideal solutions to all his problems. These false promises are designed to make the normal self of the patient dependent on or addicted to his omnipotent self, and to lure the normal sane parts into this delusional structure in order to imprison them.

(1971a: 169–78)

The converse situation can also arise and the patient may project the psychotic part of the personality into the analyst and then feel that he needs to preserve his sanity from the sadistic attacks of an analyst experienced as mad in the pursuit of his analytic task.

It is important to remember that, although the psychotic organization can come to serve as a retreat from the catastrophic anxieties of fragmentation and disintegration, even in the psychotic patient depressive feelings may emerge which are also felt to be unbearable. The delusional retreat may then be felt to be necessary in order to avoid such feelings, which may quickly be transformed and confused with those of persecution. The depressive feelings may be particularly threatening if they are felt to be an expression of the patient's sanity since they are then felt to challenge the dominance of the psychotic organization and to threaten the emergence of a dependent relationship with the analyst based on psychic reality rather than delusion.

Clinical material

I will try to illustrate some of these points with a clinical fragment from a patient, Mr C, who had recently recovered from a major breakdown, and although just able to return to work was still very paranoid and concrete in his thinking. He began a session by voicing bitter complaints against his employers who had been unfair to him and then against his analyst who did nothing to rectify this unfairness. He next described a breast infection which his mother had had when he was a baby and moved on to speak with triumph about his ability to hurt the analyst. He then announced his intention to change his job and, since this would necessitate a move to another city, it meant the end of his analysis.

The analyst felt sad at the idea of losing his patient and interpreted that the patient wanted to get rid of his own sadness and wanted *him*, the analyst, to feel the pain of separation and loss. The patient said, 'Yes, I can do to you what you do to me. You are in my hands. There is an equalization.' A moment later he started to complain that he was being poisoned and he began to discuss government policies of nuclear deterrence. He argued these were stupid because they involved total annihilation but the policies of nuclear disarmament were no better because you could not neutralize existing armaments. He then complained of gastric troubles and diarrhoea, and said he had been going to the toilet after each session recently. He explained that he had to shit out every word the analyst gave him in order not to be contaminated by infected milk.

In his response to the analyst's interpretation the patient at first appears to agree that he wants the analyst to feel the pain of separation and loss in order to effect an 'equalization', but a moment later he complains of being poisoned. I believe that he found this interpretation correct but threatening because it exposed him to experiences such as grief, anxiety, and guilt, which were associated with the loss of his analyst. He felt that the interpretation had forced him to take these feelings back into himself and he experienced them concretely as poison and tried to evacuate them in his faeces. The patient feared that this kind of experience would threaten the dominance of the psychotic organization and leave him in a desperate state. The catastrophic nature of his anxiety was indicated by the way he spoke about nuclear disaster, and his insistence that no defence was possible against a nuclear attack may have had its roots in his conviction that his defences could not protect him against the analyst's words. He needed the analyst to recognize that he could maintain a relationship with him only if the analyst agreed to hold the experiences associated with loss in his own mind and to refrain from challenging the psychotic organization by trying to return these prematurely to the patient. After a transient contact with the experience of loss the psychotic organization reasserted itself in the patient's assertion that he had been shitting out every word the analyst said.

A further clinical fragment

The nature of this patient's psychotic organization and the retreat from reality it created are illustrated in material from sessions a week or two later. An important plan which had occupied much of the analysis was the patient's intention to become a Jew, and he said he had strengthened his Jewish contacts, was learning Hebrew, and had sent off for a prayer shawl made in Israel. He had been told that circumcision was desirable but not essential and he became excited by the idea of owning a prayer shawl and spoke about David and Goliath.

He next repeated his intention to seek a job in a distant city, which meant the end of his analysis, and he became preoccupied with the idea that the analyst had a Jewish son-in-law. He complained that he had to work hard to get a Jewish identity while the analyst's daughter only had to marry a Jew. He then became increasingly abusive of the Jews in the analyst's locality who, he claimed, had a secret anti-Semitism more dangerous than the Nazis, and he also complained about the Israelis who, he believed, were delaying his prayer shawl.

When the prayer shawl finally arrived he brought it with joy and triumph to his session. He explained that the shawl gave him certainty through its link with Yahweh and if he had had it six years before, the catastrophe of his breakdown would not have happened.

The analyst interpreted that he believed that, with the help of Yahweh, he would be so powerful that he could defeat his enemies as David had defeated Goliath and that he clearly believed this was a greater source of security than he could get from his analysis.

Gradually his mood quietened, and more sadly he explained that before the breakdown he did not need such aids as the shawl. He said that then he knew how to live and he knew that 'I am I'. Something inside him had softened and dissolved. Now with the shawl he had an unconquerable power. He was glad but also sad. He usually complained about the lost time which the breakdown had cost him but now he felt he could bear that. What he could not bear was the thought that something had been lost which could never be recovered.

This rather unusual experience of contact with depressive feelings was followed by extremely violent sessions in which he claimed that he and Yahweh would destroy the world and he spoke of the annihilation of mankind. That evening he telephoned the analyst and said he was afraid he would confuse the toilet and the consulting room. He was phoning because he was afraid he would forget this fear tomorrow and he wanted the analyst to remind him. In the session he said, 'You realize that when I am enraged I will shit in your room. The disposal is your problem. They do it to me so why should I not do it to you?'

I think it is possible in the present material to see how for most of the time the patient is entrenched in a psychotic organization which serves to make him feel powerful and to restore the damage he feels has been done to his mind. The organization needs to be centred on omnipotent objects, ultimately Yahweh himself, whose support he can obtain by becoming a Jew. If the patch to the ego created by the organization is missing or delayed he is panicky and infuriated and the atmosphere becomes paranoid and is dealt with by omnipotence.

The psychotic organization which has dominated his life since his breakdown is not, however, totally in control, and depressive feelings emerge and are at first experienced in the counter-transference. The analyst feels sorry at the thought of losing his patient and is moved by the patient's longing to have an identity. The patient, however, finds such feelings of longing and dependence frightening, and I think it was this which he was afraid poisoned him as he began to recognize some of the analyst's pain, represented in a symbolic equation by the breast with an infection. He handed these feelings over to the analyst to cope with, saying, 'The disposal is your problem,' and returned to the retreat.

At the same time it is clear that the psychotic organization was a complex structure into which the analyst had been incorporated. The patient had turned to Yahweh as a source of omnipotence because he had become persuaded that he could turn the feeling of smallness and persecution into a triumph. Although the mode of expression of his longings is clearly psychotic, it is not difficult to recognize that his wish to become a Jew and many of his complaints against the analyst represent his longing to be accepted by the analyst as his son and to gain his protection and support in that way. Here the analyst is represented as a powerful Yahweh figure split off from a more ordinary, sane, but weak, analyst. The sanity of the analyst is seen as an obstacle to the achievement of these omnipotent solutions and it has either to be seduced into acquiescence or to be overwhelmed through omnipotence.

The analyst, by interpreting that with the help of Yahweh the patient wanted to be powerful and defeat his enemies, recognized the patient's need for omnipotence as a source of security. He understood that when the patient feels small and persecuted by Goliath-like figures he experiences the analyst as weak and unimpressive in what he can offer. Following this interpretation, the patient is able to acknowledge that since his breakdown he had lost a sense of identity and no longer knows that 'I am I'. He is able to express sorrow for this loss of identity which he does not believe he can ever regain and, although he is glad he has unconquerable power through the prayer shawl, he clearly wishes he could return to the state before the breakdown when he did not need such omnipotence.

Facing reality means acknowledging damage which in all probability can never be put right, and the patient, at least momentarily, can stay in touch with such painful feelings when he feels supported by an analyst who can help him mourn the loss of his capacities and his objects. Temporarily, he sounds like a disabled but sane patient, but the contact cannot be maintained and psychotic forces quickly regain control of his personality in an attempt to undo and deny the damage through omnipotence.

This patient, like the man described by Segal (1956), gave an indication that the psychotic process had not totally destroyed the capacity to feel depression and concern at his own desperate state, at the state of his objects and of his relationship with them. These moments of contact gave rise to the possibility of development and made the idea of useful analytic work seem feasible. Nevertheless, the limits to such progress and the sense of disability which he would have to accept if he faced the psychic reality of his state were also evident.

7

Revenge, resentment, remorse and reparation

An important variety of psychic retreat is one where the patient is dominated by feelings of resentment and grievance, and in this chapter I will look at the way such retreats operate as a defence against anxiety and guilt. These patients feel injured and wronged but are unable to express their wish for revenge actively by openly attacking the objects which have wronged them. Some patients are inhibited by the fear of retaliation, but in the cases I shall describe the inhibition appeared to be linked to a fear that the revenge would be excessive and would exact such retribution that the patient could not face the anxiety and guilt which would follow the realization of what he wished to do and what, in his phantasy, he had done.

The first patient, Mr D, could not acknowledge his hatred of me so that open attacks were replaced by an attitude of polite deference. He used omnipotent manic mechanisms and exacted his revenge indirectly by a restless and ruthless replacing of his objects with something new and better. In his analysis he achieved this by ignoring my interpretations and by repeatedly turning away, leaving me feeling discarded and misused. Often this appeared to be a type of revenge enacted by a reversal so that he treated me in precisely the way he felt treated both in his everyday life and in his analysis. He allied himself with an omnipotent organization which offered protection against guilt by inviting him into a manic state of mind where consideration for the state of his objects was not necessary and where damage could be undone with such omnipotence that guilt was inappropriate.

The second patient, Mr E, was less manic, and his retreat was dominated by a passivity in which he projected responsibility into his objects and waited for them to admit they were to blame. This led to a masochistic state which served to perpetuate a chronic suffering in which he felt wronged but forced to endure and to cooperate in his persecution. He occasionally realized that his hatred had damaged his objects, but he usually argued that he had no need to feel guilt. With his chronic sense of grievance he was able to feel justified and in the right.

In both patients problems became evident when they made moves to emerge from the retreat and to face their psychic reality. As they did so, they began to get a glimpse of the state their objects had been reduced to in their phantasy and they were filled with horror, and threatened with anxiety and guilt. For Mr D, such moments of contact predominantly gave rise to panic, which was chiefly associated with a time when he had been deeply depressed. He looked on the possibility of a recurrence with such dread that the slightest contact with depressive feelings sent him into a flight back to the protection of the organization. It seemed to me that the horrendous state of his objects was unconsciously felt to result from the vengeance acted out on his behalf with cruelty and ruthlessness by the organization, and also from the way he had denied any responsibility for the hatred and neglect of his objects while sheltering in the retreat. Here the pathological organization of the personality served as a protection from guilt, but as a result of its actions it also gave rise to guilt.

Mr E was less terrified of his depression, and could sometimes allow contact with an experience of loss which followed occasions when he let go of some of his resentment and passivity and was able to attack his objects more openly and actively. Such attacks were possible because he had a more secure belief that a capacity to love would survive the expression of his hatred. This capacity gave rise to feelings of responsibility, remorse and regret, which in turn stimulated a wish to make reparation.

The central issue for both patients as they attempted to free themselves from the domination of the organization was whether the guilt was bearable or not (see Steiner 1990a). If it was bearable, as was true occasionally in the case of Mr E, the patient felt able to risk a struggle for his independence from the organization, while if it was unbearable, as seemed to be the case with Mr D, the patient felt obliged to relinquish his freedom and return once more to the protection of the organization in the retreat.

In these cases pathological organizations came to be deployed in an attempt to protect the object and to evade guilt, but, in fact, only served to convert the overt attack into a more hidden and chronic campaign. The fear of a violent and open expression of hatred and destructiveness leads to a chronic state in which the object is not destroyed, or allowed to die, but is tormented, disabled, and held onto in a half dead state. Revenge is neither openly enacted nor given up.

The attempt to prevent unrestrained violence leads to an endless revenge in which there is a very intense tie to the object which must be kept alive in order that the process may continue. The patient has apparently deployed the organization to neutralize destructive elements, but the result has been only partially successful and the organization serves both to preserve the object and to enact the revenge.

Once established, this type of retreat is very difficult to relinquish partly because the grievance provides a focus and purpose for the patient and partly because of other sources of gratification such as those related to triumph and to masochism. In some cases the patient appears to 'feed' or 'nurse' the grievance and gets gratification by 'keeping old wounds open'. These expressions suggest that the resentment may be linked to early experiences such as those of weaning, or the arrival of a new baby in the family, which involved loss in a setting where this seemed unfair and the patient felt betrayed and wronged. A wound results which may become so invested with narcissism that it is denied the opportunity for proper healing. In these cases the patient may come to believe that the objects which have wronged him are so totally bad that they can never be forgiven and his own hatred and his wish for revenge are felt to be so total that they are equally unforgivable. Subsequently, even if the loss seems bearable, the injury is nursed in order to keep the sense of injustice alive and to defend against any sense of responsibility. The pathological organization supports the patient and helps him to evade guilt which is felt to be appropriate for the object rather than the patient to feel. At the same time, the conviction that the guilt is unbearable leads to an extremely stuck situation where change is resisted and progress in the analysis is blocked.

An important feature of these situations is that the patient appears to be preoccupied with the future. His current suffering is masochistically endured and he lives in hope that in the future right will be done and he will be avenged. The resentment, and with it the hope of redress, become a defence against current reality, especially against the experience of loss, and, as a result, it interferes with mourning and with development (Potamianou 1992). When a sense of grievance and hatred dominates, the psychic reality of the patient's internal relationships reflects the fact that destructive attacks have already taken place and continue to be enacted as long as the hatred and the wish for revenge remain alive. The very existence of hatred towards the object means that, in phantasy, attacks have been mounted and that the object has already been damaged. Evidence of these attacks may appear in dreams, fantasies and other material but, in the psychic retreat, either their existence or their significance is denied. As long as the hatred goes unacknowledged, attacks can continue without any sense of responsibility, guilt or conflict.

Nevertheless, for brief periods, at least in some cases, the patient is able to emerge from the retreat so that the torturing becomes less prominent and his impulses towards the object are more open and direct. If he can retain sufficient contact with his psychic reality to acknowledge both his hatred, which leads to the wish to destroy the object, and his love, which makes him feel remorse and regret, then development can proceed. The contact with the reality of the state of his objects allows him to recognize the damage his hatred has accomplished, and he is able to struggle with those rich and painful experiences connected with loss which we associate with mourning. As mourning is worked through projective identification is reversed and the subject is able to regain parts of the self previously disowned (see Chapter 5). Feelings of *remorse* and *guilt* arise, and the capacity to endure, suffer and survive these experiences leads to a shift towards the depressive position in which loss is acknowledged and attempts at making reparation can begin to evolve. In other patients any contact with an object which has been damaged in phantasy leads to panic and an immediate return to the psychic retreat.

Clinical material

The first patient, Mr D, worked as a research fellow in a cut-throat academic climate where rivalry was at times deadly. He habitually entered new situations with a flourish and made a promising start which eventually led to disappointment. He became seriously depressed at university when he was first promoted and later sacked as an editor of a student newspaper, and he feared a recurrence of the depression and sought analysis chiefly to avert such an eventuality. In fact, the situation at his work was becoming increasingly precarious partly because he could not bear criticism, so that numerous clashes with his superiors led to a furious reaction which he had to suppress to ensure his survival.

His personal involvement in the rivalry was denied, as too was his jealousy of an older sister who was not academic and was married with a young baby. He recognized the pleasure which his sister gave his parents but saw this as something which he would easily surpass as soon as he was able to bring off his research success and with its aid acquire the kind of wife his parents would approve of.

77

A great deal of time was spent planning moves to different departments, to different countries and even to different fields of research, and although in fantasy these led to triumph over his colleagues and teachers, he did not see them as vengeful and he denied any hatred towards those who constantly appeared to overlook his importance and to prevent his advancement.

He began a session by describing a meeting which took place in the office next door to his on the previous day. It was in the Senior Lecturer's room and he was not invited, which rubbed in the fact that he no longer had a place in the department. Later he had a serious talk with the Senior Lecturer who gave him advice about how to handle himself better. He was told that he made impulsive decisions which were not to be trusted, and the patient responded compliantly by agreeing that this was absolutely correct and by expressing gratitude for what the department had done for him. In fact, it was clear from his frequent disparaging remarks about this lecturer and about the department that he thought of himself as superior and that he was holding his tongue until he could show them all how he would succeed in a different setting.

He went on to speak excitedly, but with some lack of conviction, about his new prospects and research plans, but he added that he thought I would be disappointed in him since I would view these as a repetition of a cycle and see him as 'back to square one'. He went on to say that he noticed that he did not tell me things any more, as if the analysis was also virtually over. For example, on Friday he had asked a particularly attractive new girl to go out with him but he added that he was a little disappointed in her lack of enthusiasm. He had broken off the relationship with his old girl-friend more than a year before but continued to phone her and discussed his new jobs and new girls with her in great detail. Now he complained that he had left a message for her and she had failed to phone him back. He wondered if it was because he had recently spoken about his masturbation, which had come up in the analysis. She had said, 'How disgusting', or was it 'How pathetic'? He said it was unlike her to be disgusted with another person's misery.

I interpreted that he was afraid I was put off by the way he was discussing his plans to leave his job and also his analysis. His excitement with new jobs as well as his plans for new girls were spoken about in the session as if they did not involve me, just as the Senior Lecturer held meetings in his office without including him. Now he was afraid I was just like an ex-girl-friend and that he was back to square one. He had begun the analysis with enthusiasm but he now felt so hurt and wronged that it had become intolerable.

78

His reaction was to say that he sees all that but he has to do it and he is sure that I understand. I interpreted that he hoped that I could see that he felt he had no choice, and that he was obliged to dismiss what I said to him as unimportant just as he was forced to turn to other departments, which meant the end of the analysis and felt like a return to square one. I suggested that the underlying situation which he could not bear was one in which the meeting held in the next-door office reminded him of my independent existence and of times when he was excluded. This was particularly acute when a holiday or weekend was impending as was now the case, since I had given him my holiday dates in the previous session.

He said that he felt I hated it when he became arrogant and dismissive of me, and I think he sensed that I was affected and vulnerable. However, he added that when I spoke about things like holidays it had no effect on him and he assumed that he had a blind spot since he never understood why I took that up so often. He found that his mind turned to other things. He did not feel any hostility to me although he thought I was right and that he hated the Senior Lecturer, the Professor and also his father. I interpreted that, although he was staying calm and superior, he was upset when he felt I was disappointed in him. I think he saw me as someone who had to protect himself and that I became superior in turn and tried to make him feel dependent on the analysis.

Although fantasies of a triumphant reversal of his dependence on his father, on his professors and on his girl-friend were quite conscious and he could recognize that this involved turning the tables on them, he did not admit that he felt any hatred and he did not connect these fantasies with a wish for revenge. Nor was he able to acknowledge his hatred of the analysis, which he consciously saw as something he valued and was simply forced to give up due to circumstances. That I persevered with interpretations about weekends and breaks was something he tolerantly put up with. The violence which an open revenge would involve was replaced by the cruelty of his withdrawal to a psychic retreat in which I was deemed too unimportant even to attack. He kept me imprisoned and obliged to listen while he described his plans for new relationships which would exclude me. He spoke as if I was tolerant and understanding, but I think he had at least a partial realization that I was often provoked to feel irritated and resentful.

Two sessions later he began with a discussion of some entrepreneurial projects which involved selling some of his research ideas to a group of industrialists, and he then described an interview he had with a professor at a polytechnic who was thinking of offering him a job which turned out to be at a considerably lower level than he expected. He would not accept that level but he thought he would play them off against another department which he was more likely to join. He said that he did not want to burn his bridges as he had with a previous attempt to leave his post. He was also continuing the stand-off relationship with his father after the incident with his sister's baby. At a family celebration he had given the baby a sip of champagne as a joke and his father had been angry, especially emphasizing that it was not his baby so that he had no right to decide what to give him. He had to suppress his anger but reacted by rejecting a dinner invitation from his mother.

Through the thought of burning his bridges, he came closer to making contact with a fear that I would not want him back as he repeatedly destroyed my goodwill with his various triumphant plans. I thought this might have led to a momentary experience of loss which made him panic. After a second or two he returned to his previous mood with a description of how he and another girl-friend had laughed at the interview he had had at the polytechnic. The Head of Department was a typical 'poly' type, with narrow views. It would have been a job with a lot of teaching and almost no research, a 9–5 office job, with no excitement and no inventiveness. In this instance emergence from the retreat could not be tolerated and he returned to his triumphant mania.

The second patient, Mr E, had, in many ways, made good use of his analysis and was successful in his work and increasingly contented in his marriage. In the analysis situations sometimes arose which provoked 'bad' thoughts, and in the past these had often made him feel that he was all bad, and that he could not be forgiven. As an infant he had, in fact, been left to cry for long periods when his mother was depressed, and I thought that he must have felt so full of badness and that he had created such worry and despair that he was convinced that his mother and now myself did not want him and would leave him to die.

He usually dealt with the panic which resulted from this sort of situation by idealizing his logic and thinking and getting reassurance that he was wanted by having it valued and admired. If I did not agree to this he felt that I was denying his goodness and sentencing him to feel so bad that he could not believe I could want him at all. When I failed to provide reassurance through admiration it meant that I disliked him, blamed him for *my* depression and wished him dead. This used to fill him with hatred and led to further 'bad' thoughts. If I admired him, however, he felt that he had been able to enlist me to

80

collude with in an organization which helped him to deny his
aggression and destructiveness. In the retreat, the idealization and the
grievance both appeared to be supported by the same organization, and
the resentment came to be focused on my refusal to join in the
idealization.

There was a particular quality to his reaction to some of my failures
and shortcomings. I had clearly done something bad which excluded
him, and made him feel disliked and unwanted, but there was, in
addition, a sense of betrayal which gave a particular edge to his
indignation and outrage. I was made to feel that I had done something
unpardonable which put me beyond the pale and disqualified me so
that I became someone unfit to be a psychoanalyst. It was not that he
found me to be a mixture of good and bad elements; I was all bad and
had to be shown as such. These situations were very unpleasant and he
often succeeded in undermining my confidence in my work and in my
integrity, particularly when I had reason to feel bad about something I
had done or failed to do. They were accompanied by an offer of a way
out. If I would agree to a collusive and defensive idealization, everything would be put right.

One day he began a session saying that he had felt a bit uncomfortable as he entered the building. The waiting room felt somewhat
strange and he noticed that I sneezed as I came down to get him. He
hoped I was not getting a cold and realized I had been under strain
recently. I had in fact taken a week off which he knew was because of
a bereavement a couple of weeks previously.

He went on to say that he had a reasonably good week-end, most of
which he spent at a party political congress, in his function as a political
journalist. While restless on Saturday, he had many dreams but could
only remember one fragment. He had placed a piece of faeces in a gift
box as a present for someone. People were commenting on this and
someone said it was a result of anxiety. Someone else said it was his
wish to spoil and make a mess of things.

He thought the dream had to do with the congress and he
connected it with feelings of rivalry with colleagues. He then remembered his feelings of hurt in the session on Friday when I had
interpreted his use of logic as an idealized production which disguised what he really felt. This had reminded him of previous
occasions when he had felt extremely persecuted by me. At these
times he felt that everything he tried to bring me was rebuffed, and
he would panic that there was nothing he could talk about which I
would find acceptable.

He proceeded to go back to talk about the congress where he met a friend who told him that a Member of Parliament he had worked with had been dangerously ill. He had known nothing of the illness and had indeed repeatedly telephoned this man, putting pressure on him to provide him with some data which he needed for an article. His first thought was of anxiety and regret but this was quickly replaced by what he called a 'shitty' thought; namely, that the MP's illness served him right for refusing to help him.

I thought he felt bad about his reaction to my recent week off, and not knowing any details made him feel excluded and de-manding. The 'shitty' thought towards the MP had a parallel with the thought that, because I had excluded him, I deserved all that I got. However, he also saw that I had not quite recovered from my bereavement, and he was sorry and had enough good feeling to recognize the thought as 'shitty'.

I interpreted that he still felt bad about his 'shitty' thought, but not so bad as he previously did because he also felt he had good feelings of regret and sorrow when he gave me a difficult time. This meant that he was not in the same panic as he used to get into, but he was still unsure if he could admit it as a bad thought or if he needed to wrap it up as something good. He still wanted me to reassure him that the hostile thought was not really a bad one because it was so well wrapped up and was anyhow a result of anxiety. This meant that he could not be blamed, and if I did not agree it could easily lead to my becoming the bad figure who hated him unjustly. I connected this with the uncertainty in the dream as to whether the faeces were brought out of anxiety, perhaps as an infantile gift to cure a depressed mother, or out of a wish to spoil. He responded by saying that he also felt rebuffed when he took so much trouble to do something for me which I then failed to appreciate.

It seemed clear that when he felt so humiliated he was convinced that he would not be accepted and this led to anxiety even amounting to terror, because to be hated was equated with being cast out and left to die. Now the situation seemed to have changed, and it was no longer so clear that he could not bear these experiences. If he could admit the idea that he wanted to exact revenge and to do so by spoiling my work, it made guilt available and this in turn could lead to regret and a wish to make reparation. This wish to spoil was particularly intense when he felt that his efforts to put things right by bringing gifts was frustrated by my failure to recognize the good qualities mixed in with his hatred.

Discussion

Both of the patients I have discussed harboured resentments about wrongs which they felt were done to them and which continued to be done to them. Although the two patients were very different in terms of their mental make-up and the defences which they used, they both harboured grievances and could not free themselves from them to become conscious of their wish to damage their objects. In fact when they withdrew in grievance to the psychic retreat, their hatred, although perhaps less manifestly violent, remained extremely powerful as it slowly and more secretly poisoned their relationships and drew them towards self-destructive acts.

Each made moves to emerge from their retreat and made at least transient contact with the psychic reality confronting them. In the case of Mr D I thought this occurred when he presumed I would view him as 'back to square one', and again when he became afraid that he had 'burnt his bridges'. These instances seemed to represent moments when the patient felt threatened by a loss and which led him to panic and to return abruptly to a manic superiority. It was as if he believed that any experience of loss would throw him into the depression he dreaded. Mr E was able to sustain the contact with loss for a longer period and could acknowledge his hatred for the Member of Parliament and his wish to get even with him. Moreover, he could make a connection with similar wishes towards his analyst and could recognize what he called 'shitty thoughts'. This enabled him to make some progress towards accepting loss and making reparation. However, even here the contact could not be prolonged and a constant movement between withdrawal to the retreat and an emergence from it continued.

Both patients faced that critical point in the depressive position, described in Chapter 3, which arises when the task of relinquishing control over the object has to be faced. As long as they held onto their grievance the object was possessed and controlled, so that they remained stuck in the first phase of the depressive position in which loss is denied. This phase has to be overcome if the depressive position is to be worked through and the object is to be allowed its independence. Klein (1935) described the situation as fundamental for understanding 'the loss of the loved object'; namely, that situation when 'the ego becomes fully identified with its good internalised objects, and at the same time becomes aware of its own incapacity to protect and preserve them against the internalised persecuting objects and the id' (p. 265). Some patients are able to relinquish omnipotent control over their objects, to allow them to go, and to face the fact that in psychic reality this means to allow them to die. Others panic and return to the protection of the retreat.

Winnicott (1969, 1971) discusses this problem when he differentiates between what he calls *relating* to an object and what he calls *use* of an object. In this particular meaning of 'relating to an object' the patient omnipotently possesses and controls the object through what Klein calls projective identification. In order to relinquish such control and to enable the object to be 'placed outside the area of subjective phenomena', Winnicott argues that the object has to be destroyed by the subject. Then, when the external object returns, having survived the attacks, a new type of relationship becomes possible – 'the use of an object', namely, one in which the object is real and recognized to be outside the patient's omnipotent control (Winnicott 1971: 90).

Unfortunately, the reappearance of the object which has survived the attacks can also be used to deny the reality of the attacks and to reassure the patient that there is no need for remorse or guilt. When this happens, the object's survival has served to help the patient evade the psychic reality with which the patient had made transient contact. In other cases, the patient realizes that the object, even though it has survived the attacks, remains damaged in the patient's psychic reality, and its return does not remove the fact that there had been a wish to destroy it. At the same time the patient's omnipotent belief that the fate of his object lies entirely in his hands must also be relinquished as the reality of the object's independence is appreciated. Guilt has to be faced, and this must be appropriate to what has been lost. The loss has to be acknowledged and mourned, and this includes the loss of the patient's omnipotence. If the analyst can resist acting out, either through retaliation or through collusion, he can support the patient and help him to survive the situation in his internal world. In particular, he can help him get the events in proportion and in many circumstances can help him to locate positive feelings which can come to mitigate his hatred. It is these loving feelings, together with the acknowledgement of the destructive wishes, which enable reparation to be pursued.

In this context reparation often takes the form of forgiveness, since for the relationship to be repaired the patient has to feel able to forgive and also to be forgiven. If he is to change and to allow development, he has ultimately to forgive his objects for the wrongs they have inflicted and he can only do this if he is convinced that he himself is forgiven for what *he* has done and for what he wished to do. Rey is one of the few analysts to discuss this aspect of reparation. He describes how his clinical experience has led him to consider that forgiveness is a key concept.

[F]or nobody who has not forgiven can be expected to *feel* forgiven. This leads to desire of revenge towards the object to remain active and therefore the feeling that the object still seeks revenge and has not forgiven. . . . Only when the super-ego becomes less cruel, less demanding as well of perfection, is the ego capable of accepting an internal object which is not perfectly repaired, can accept compromise, forgive and be forgiven, and experience hope and gratitude.

(Rey 1986: 30)

Forgiveness requires us to recognize the coexistence of good and bad feelings, sufficient badness to justify guilt, and sufficient goodness to deserve forgiveness. We need to believe this is true of ourselves and also of our objects. The wish to exact revenge must be recognized, and responsibility for the damage we have done to our objects has to be accepted. This means that to be forgiven, bad elements in our nature have to be accepted but sufficient good feeling must exist for us to feel regret and to wish to make reparation.

In the cases I have described the central issue seemed to be that the patients felt that I had done something unforgivable, and this led me to the question of why it was that the patient could not forgive. I came to the conclusion that revenge is a complex phenomenon. It often appears to begin with a real or imagined wrong which provokes no more than a wish for justice and a reasonable compensation. The demand for revenge is particularly pressing when the injury and wrong has been done not only to the self but also to good internal objects which are represented by the family or group. The conscious aim of the revenge may then be to clear the good name of the injured object and to restore the family honour. Revenge here begins as an expression of the life instinct, and demands that we stand up against those who injure us and threaten our objects.

In practice, justice is seldom able to intervene in an adequate way, and its failure to give satisfaction allows other motives to become attached to the initially just cause. Old hatreds, based on narcissistic wounds, greed, jealousy, Oedipal rivalries, and especially the primitive destructiveness rooted in envy, take over and give revenge its insatiable nature, with devastating consequences if it is not restrained. When the death instinct comes to dominate, revenge is not satisfied until the object and with it the self is totally destroyed.

These characteristics make the open expression of revenge dangerous because it gives rise to a fear of retribution from a stronger object or a fear of guilt if the revenge were to be successfully and excessively carried through. The patient is trapped in a deadly internal situation where he feels wronged and unable to gain redress. His withdrawal to the psychic retreat has offered him the protection of a complex network of object relations often involving powerful and ruthlessly destructive objects functioning as a Mafia-like gang. Such gangs are expert in revenge and gain a hold over the patient by promising the eventual destruction of his enemies (Rosenfeld 1971a).

The operation of the pathological organization takes place in a phantasy world, sometimes partly conscious but carefully prevented from being openly enacted. The external situation is carefully preserved, but in phantasy the attack leads to such devastation that its consequences are too horrible to be faced. The sense of guilt which this generates becomes unbearable, and is dealt with by projective identification so that it comes to reside in the object where it becomes indistinguishable from the object's own badness. The result is that the patient is confronted by an object which is so bad that it cannot be forgiven and which must not be let off the hook but must be punished or destroyed. It is important, however, to understand that from the patient's point of view it is the analyst who seems to be unable to admit his badness and to face his guilt. The patient experiences the situation as a repetitive one where badness is attributed to him by his objects, who demand that he accept it and put right what is felt to be the object's fault. It is sometimes crucial for the patient to see that the analyst is able to examine his contribution to the impasse and to face a guilt which is appropriate to what he has done.

As with so many themes in psychoanalysis, the outcome of the conflict depends on the balance between life and death instincts, between love and hate, between good and evil. Ultimately it is the fear that hatred dominates which prevents the acknowledgements of guilt and which favours omnipotent solutions.

My patient, Mr D, was not convinced that he had sufficient good feelings to risk the acknowledgement of his vengeful impulses and to protect his objects from the enactment of the revenge. His relationship to an internal source of goodness was insecure, and this led him to panic when he became aware of his hatred of his objects. He felt obliged to project the badness and have it denied by omnipotent, manic pseudo-reparation. Mr E had a greater belief in a source of internal goodness with which he could identify so that, for example, the gift of faeces could be recognized as one showing intense ambivalence. This led at least to a transient belief that he could be forgiven and lessened the need to deny his hatred and his destructive, 'shitty' thoughts. Such developments are always insecure, and further cycles of emergence from the retreat followed by a return to it inevitably recur. However, as these become repeatedly acted out in the relationship with the analyst, a greater capacity to recognize the damage done can arise and periods of contact with depressive feelings become increasingly possible.

8

The relationship to reality in psychic retreats

We have seen how a psychic retreat comes to represent a place where respite from anxiety is sought and that this is achieved by a greater or lesser divorce from contact with reality. In some psychotic retreats the rupture with reality may be extreme, but in most retreats a special relationship with reality is established in which reality is neither fully accepted nor completely disavowed. I believe that this constitutes a third type of relation to reality, which I will describe in this chapter, and which contributes to the fixed character of the retreat. It is related to mechanisms similar to those which Freud described in the case of fetishism (1927) and which play an important part in perversion.

Rigidity results if projected parts of the self cannot be withdrawn from objects and returned to the ego and, as we have seen – for example, in Chapter 5 – this task requires a capacity to face reality in order that mourning can proceed. Even if partial contact is achieved, evasion is often sufficient to prevent the acceptance of loss and consequently to interfere with the working through of mourning. The retreat in this way leads to an evasion of the experience of loss, and mourning proceeds only to the first stage where objects are possessed rather than relinquished. Projections are consequently not withdrawn from the object to be returned to the self and the only way of retaining contact with lost parts of the self is through a possessive hold on the object into which they have been projected. The original rigidity of the pathological organizations of the personality is consequently unaltered through experience.

This may not be too serious if the respite from reality is partial and transient but problems arise when it becomes long-term or permanent. The retreat may become so regular a feature that it is no longer a transient shelter but more a way of life, and the patient may come to inhabit a kind of dream or fantasy world which he finds preferable to the real world.

Although we usually associate the word 'perversion' with sexual perversions, it has become increasingly recognized that the concept has a wider reference. Some contemporary analysts (Chasseguet-Smirgel 1974, 1981, 1985; McDougall 1972) have come to emphasize the way in which reality is misrepresented in the perversions, and others (Money-Kyrle 1968; Joseph 1989; Britton *et al.* 1989) have described perverse distortions in areas other than the sexual. These developments can be seen as a reflection of the state of mind where reality is simultaneously accepted and disavowed.

Most dictionary definitions of the words 'perverse' and 'perversion' have emphasized the theme of 'turning away from the truth'. Thus the *Shorter Oxford English Dictionary* (1933) defines 'perverse' as '*Turned away from what is right*'. In legal usage it refers to a verdict which is '*against the weight of evidence or the direction of the judge*' and it also implies a certain wilfulness. Thus a second definition is '*Obstinate or persistent in what is wrong; self-willed or stubborn*' and '*Disposed to be obstinately contrary to what is true or good or to go counter to what is reasonable or required*'. The definition of 'perversion' is similar, and reminds us that in a religious context it is the opposite of 'conversion'. The definition of the verb 'to pervert' includes the idea of corruption or leading astray away from a right opinion or action. It is interesting that, except in more recent editions, the idea of perversion as a deviant sexual act is missing or only briefly mentioned, and it struck me that in our current thinking on perverse mechanisms we are turning more to the lay dictionary meaning of the term and seeing sexual perversion as a special instance of a more general perverse attitude to what is true and right.

In addition to the issue of turning away from what is right, there are two overtones discernible in the definitions which are important in analysis. First, there is a degree of wilfulness, obstinacy, or stubbornness assumed, which suggests that the pervert is not without insight into what is right and wrong, or conflict about which path to choose. The wilfulness implies that, in part at least, he knows what is true and right and that nevertheless he turns away from it. I will argue that he both knows and does not know, and that it is the way in which these two attitudes are simultaneously held and yet apparently reconciled which is characteristic of perversion.

Second, there is the suggestion, at least in the transitive verb 'to pervert', that someone is perverted, led astray, or corrupted by an agency working against what is true and right. I will later try to show how in pathological organizations of the personality various alliances are formed, leading to complex collusions between forces which are often experienced as representatives of good and evil. The patient often feels himself to be a victim of pressure to which he is obliged to submit.

In perversion such submission may have an element of insight attached to it and the victim may not be as helpless as he at first seems. This theme is examined in the next chapter (Chapter 9), where I look at the perverse character of the retreat from the point of view of the object relations involved. The structure of pathological organizations of the personality will be emphasized, and I will describe how members of the narcissistic gang which comprise the organization are held together by perverse types of interaction in which sadism often plays a prominent role.

The nature of perversion has been much discussed and I will not attempt a review here. Most writers have emphasized Freud's early views in which he described infantile sexuality as 'polymorphously perverse'. Clinical perversion was then considered to be simply the persistence into adulthood of these infantile patterns which in perversion, in contrast to neurosis, fail to be repressed. It is this notion which gave rise to the famous and rather misleading dictum that 'neuroses are so to say the negative of perversions' (Freud 1905b). Freud later made it clear (1919), and most writers agree, that perversion, like neurosis, is a compromise formed from the conflict between impulse, defence, and anxiety. In 'A child is being beaten' (1919) he emphasizes the anxieties of the Oedipus complex and sees the sado-masochistic phantasies as a defence against these anxieties.

These and other studies are ably reviewed by Gillespie (1956, 1964), who discusses the influential paper by Sachs (1923) on this theme where he suggested that the ego makes a kind of bargain with the id and allows certain perverse acts to remain ego-syntonic in exchange for which the id agrees to a repression of the bulk of infantile sexuality, particularly those aspects associated with the Oedipus complex.

Glasser (1979, 1985), Laufer and Laufer (1984), Socarides (1978), Khan (1979), and Stoller (1975), all emphasize the defensive function of perversions, the relationship to Oedipal anxieties, and the important role of eroticization of object relations. The misrepresentation of reality in perversion is mentioned by Gillespie (1964), but it remains for the French analysts, especially Chasseguet-Smirgel (1974, 1981, 1985) and McDougall (1972), to give it a central place in the study of perversion. They discuss the pervert's relation to reality, in particular the reality of the difference between the sexes and between the generations, and argue that a perverse world is created in which this reality is distorted and misrepresented.

I believe that these misrepresentations are central to an understanding of perversions and that they arise from a quite specific mechanism in which contradictory versions of reality are allowed to coexist simultaneously. This is a mechanism described very clearly by Freud in his studies of fetishism (1927), which, however, is of more general application than Freud realized and is central not only to all the sexual perversions but to the operation of perverse mechanisms in other areas also. This mechanism is characteristic of the operation of pathological organizations of the personality, and operates in many types of psychic shelter where a retreat from reality is provided while at the same time a degree of contact with reality is permitted.

Freud's discussion of fetishism

Our understanding of the way in which reality is misrepresented in perversion was initiated by Freud's discussion of fetishism (1927). Freud thought that the idea of not having a penis is associated with castration and that the boy fears that if his mother can lose her penis he might lose his. He suggested that the fetish was a substitute for the woman's penis that the little boy once believed in, and that he does not want to give up this belief in the face of the evidence of material reality.

It is clear that Freud's theme goes much deeper than the specific question of fetishism and concerns the individual's relationship with reality. Freud begins the discussion of the question (1923) by suggesting that a powerful assumption held by the child as he comes to face reality is that no difference between the sexes exists. To bring such a belief into line with reality the child's perception of the world has to lead to a relinquishment of the original theory, and Freud shows how this achievement may require the overcoming of enormous resistance. He introduces the very important idea that the child's belief which arises from his assumption and the belief arising from observation may coexist. I believe that this coexistence leads to a third type of relationship with reality characteristic of perversion and typically deployed in pathological organizations of the personality.

Freud, in an earlier paper, writes as follows:

> We know how children react to their first impressions of the absence of a penis. They disavow the fact and believe that they *do* see a penis, all the same. They gloss over the contradiction between observation and preconception by telling themselves that the penis is still small and will grow bigger presently.
>
> (1923: 143)

This point is elaborated in the famous paper on fetishism:

> It is not true that, after the child has made his observation of the woman, he has preserved unaltered his belief that women have a phallus. *He has retained that belief but he has also given it up.* In the

91

conflict between the weight of the unwelcome perception and the force of his counter-wish a compromise has been reached as is only possible under the dominance of the unconscious laws of thought – the primary process. Yes, in his mind the woman *has* got a penis in spite of everything, but this penis is no longer the same as it was before... Something else [the fetish] has taken its place.

(Freud 1927: 154; italics are mine)

Again, in 1940, he makes a similar point, as follows:

His [earlier] sight of the female genital might have convinced our child of that possibility. But he drew no such conclusion from it, since his disinclination to doing so was too great and there was no motive present which could compel him to. On the contrary, whatever uneasiness he may have felt was calmed by the reflection that what was missing would yet make its appearance: she would grow one (a penis) later. . . .

This way of dealing with reality, *which almost deserves to be described as artful*, was decisive as regards the boy's practical behaviour. He continued with his masturbation as though it implied no danger to his penis; but at the same time, in complete contradiction to his apparent boldness or indifference, he developed a symptom which showed that he nevertheless did recognize the danger.

(Freud 1940: 276–7; italics are mine)

Here Freud is discussing a sexual perversion and the fact of life which the child finds difficult to accept emerges from his observation that women do not have a penis. This is one of the central facts which establish the existence of a difference between the sexes and can be thought of as one of the *facts of life*. I will follow Money–Kyrle (1968) and argue that there are other facts of life which meet a similar fate and which also tend to be dealt with by a simultaneous acceptance and disavowal. In this context it is interesting to note that in the paper on fetishism Freud gives two examples, neither of which have anything to do with a female penis or with fetishism. His patients were both unable to face the reality of the death of their father. He wrote:

But further research led to another solution of the difficulty. It turned out that the two young men had no more 'scotomised' their father's death than a fetishist does the castration of women. It was only one current of their mental life that had not recognized their father's death; there was another current which took full account of that fact. The attitude which fitted in with the wish and the attitude which fitted in with reality existed side by side.

(Freud 1927: 156)

Earlier, in the course of a discussion of children's ideas of death, he quoted another example, in a quite different context, as follows:

> I was astonished to hear a highly intelligent boy of ten remark after the sudden death of his father: 'I know father's dead, but what I can't understand is why he doesn't come home to supper.'
>
> (Freud 1900: 254)

Here he seems to recognize how difficult it is for the child to come to terms with the meaning of death and that a compromise is to acknowledge it and deny it simultaneously. The reality of death is another of *the facts of life* and is also subject to misrepresentation by the persistence of contradictory views. Of course it does not follow that the boy in this example was being perverse because the two versions of his father were still split off from each other. It would, however, be perverse to try to reconcile them in an 'artful' way; for example, to persuade the boy that his father *will* come to supper one day, or will come if he is good. The perverse aim is to protect the child from having to face reality rather than to help him confront it.

It should be stressed that it is not simply the coexistence of contradiction which is perverse, because such a contradiction may after all result, at a more primitive level, from a splitting of the ego. The perversion arises as integration begins, and lies in the attempt to find a false reconciliation between the contradictory views which become difficult to keep separate as integration proceeds. Such a reconciliation is not necessary when splitting keeps the contradictory views totally separate and unable to influence each other. The problem only arises as the split begins to lessen and an attempt is made to integrate the two views.

It is then that three options become relevant. Either,

1 The wished-for assumption gives way to reality leading to mental pain and anxiety, which can ultimately lead, via the reality principle, to mental health; or

2 the observation of reality is nullified, or the perceptual apparatus itself is attacked, leading to a survival of the assumption and a destruction of the observation which contradicted it; this is the psychotic option; or

3 the belief based on the assumption and that based on observation are simultaneously maintained as they had been while the split was intact. Now, however, because of the integration they have to be reconciled and it is here that the perverse argument is introduced. Insight is available but is now used to misrepresent reality. It is this mechanism which Freud referred to as 'artful' and which I believe is

perverse. In Chapter 10 I discuss 'turning a blind eye' as a means of knowingly deciding not to know and I relate it to Freud's ideas on fetishism. This is one of the ways in which contradictory versions of reality are able to coexist and it is often a feature of psychic retreats.

It is interesting to note that a resort to perverse mechanisms arises in the course of development precisely because of the trend towards integration which begins to put a strain on the ego. Something similar happens in analysis when progress leads to a move towards integration. The patient may have previously been able to keep idealized and persecutory versions of himself, and of his objects, apart but finds that, as treatment proceeds, he gains insight, and can no longer do this. A stage is commonly reached when he can no longer maintain the split but does not yet feel able to tolerate the reality which integration brings. Perverse mechanisms then become accentuated and may lead to a stalemate if the patient is rescued by a pathological organization of the personality which provides a retreat or shelter in which the perverse reconciliation of opposites is allowed.

The facts of life

This perverse relationship to reality leads not so much to evasion as to misrepresentation and distortion of the truth, and Money-Kyrle came to regard these misrepresentations as a central obstacle to progress in analysis. He wrote as follows:

> my dominant assumption is that *The patient, whether clinically ill or not, suffers from unconscious misconceptions and delusions*. . . . Where, for example, I would formerly have interpreted a patient's dream as a representation of the parents' intercourse, I would now more often interpret it as a misrepresentation of this event. Indeed, every conceivable representation of it seems to proliferate in the unconscious *except the right one*.
>
> (Money-Kyrle 1968: 417)

In his later paper, Money-Kyrle (1971) suggests that he now conceptualizes the aim of analysis to be to 'help the patient understand, and so overcome, emotional impediments to his discovering what he innately already knows'. Elsewhere (Steiner 1990a), I have elaborated his argument to suggest that it is such misrepresentations of reality which are the chief obstacle when we attempt to help the patient come to terms with the reality of loss. This reality has to be faced if mourning is to proceed and projective identification is to be reversed.

Money-Kyrle proposes that all adult thinking, all later acts of recognition, are hampered by the difficulties which beset the recognition of a few fundamental aspects of reality, and of these primal *facts of life* he considers three to be supremely important. They are aspects of reality which seem particularly difficult to accept and without which no adequate acceptance of other aspects of reality is possible. His three primal facts of life consist of: 'the recognition of the breast as a supremely good object, the recognition of the parents' intercourse as a supremely creative act, and the recognition of the inevitability of time and ultimately death' (1971: 443). I believe all three are vital for the experience of the reality of loss and all have powerful defences mounted against their recognition.

The first fact, 'the recognition of the breast as the supremely good object', is a poetic way of expressing the fundamental truth that the chief source of goodness required for the infant's survival resides outside him in the external world. The wishful belief which is held onto with such resistance arises from the narcissistic defence, based on the belief that it is the infant who creates the good object which resides within him and is under his control. If bad early experiences predominate over good ones, as in the case of severely traumatized or deprived children, this narcissistic defence is even more pronounced. It is difficult for the child to recognize that even when his mother has deprived and damaged him she has also often been the source of what available goodness there was. Reality is felt as a blow to this narcissism, and when it cannot be evaded a narcissistic wound with the associated resentment results.

Under the heading of this fact of life come all the problems of the early infant's recognition of his dependence on his mother. The breast comes to symbolize and stand for the external source of everything good and the narcissistic defence deals with the problem by taking over the breast and evading any experience of separateness.

In the paranoid–schizoid position, perverse mechanisms are not required to deal with this problem because splitting ensures that good and bad experiences are kept separate. The infant associates only good experiences with the good breast because any frustration or disappointment is split off and connected with a completely different object, the bad breast. It is particularly Bion (1962a) who described how the absence of the good object is experienced concretely as the presence of the bad object in the inner world. At the paranoid–schizoid level of functioning the facts of life are dealt with by splitting and omnipotent control. The infant can retain the delusion that he *is* the good breast, or that he possesses the good breast since all experience of the contrary is associated with a split-off, persecuting relationship with the bad

95

breast. No perverse reconciliation is required as long as the split ensures that no contact between the good and the bad is allowed.

When integration begins the good and the bad objects come to be recognized as one and the same, and ultimately this will lead to a degree of acceptance of reality and a move towards the depressive position. As this is worked through, projective identification lessens and separateness between self and object is increasingly acknowledged so that the relationship becomes less narcissistic. Reality therefore comes to bear on two related distinctions, that between the good and bad objects and that between self and object. The breast is recognized not to be all good, but its goodness is seen to belong to it and not to be a creation of the subject.

Often, however, this integration turns out to be too threatening and a third relationship with reality is adopted – that is, the perverse one. Integration is neither accepted nor totally denied. Splitting lessens but the contradiction persists and becomes a problem. It is then that a perverse justification for simultaneously retaining the contradictory views provides a way out.

In relation to the first fact of life the patient comes to recognize that not all the goodness he experiences comes from within him or is under his control. This leads him to accept the existence of a good external object, but his acceptance is not complete and he simultaneously agrees to deny it. In analysis we sometimes see this when the patient attends regularly with a general appreciation of the value of the analysis, which is recognized as good. At the same time he rejects every interpretation given him, none of which seems to reflect the goodness he believes to be there. The patient often reconciles this contradiction by an 'artful' kind of explanation such as, 'the analyst secretly agrees with me that I am special but is forced for professional reasons to treat me like the other patients'.

This is not the place to discuss narcissistic defences which have been extensively studied by many authors, some of whose work I have touched on in Chapter 4. It is clear that a number of anxieties arise if the reality of the external source of goodness is recognized and these are all aspects of the experience of separateness. Perhaps the most powerfully disabling consequence of such separateness is the arousal of envy, and this may be the most potent factor maintaining the narcissistic defence. If we are searching for a term analogous to 'sexual perversion' to describe this type of misrepresentation of reality, perhaps *'narcissistic perversion'* might suit.

Money-Kyrle's second fact of life consists of 'the recognition of the parents' intercourse as a supremely creative act', and is also a poetic formulation. It is his way of introducing the problems associated with the recognition of the primal scene and the Oedipus complex. The intrusion of a third object into the baby–mother relationship introduces new problems and new questions. Jealousy is provoked, and the issue of creativity is symbolized by the child's curiosity about where babies come from.

When these anxieties are successfully negotiated, the child comes to recognize the creativity of the parental couple and through identification with them can embark on his own creative life, including that of sexual relationships. If he cannot relinquish his parents and needs to participate in their sexual relationship he remains stuck, as if symbolically or sometimes actually unable to leave home.

Various defences are mounted to deal with the painful experience of feeling excluded from the primal couple, and again projective identification is deployed as a defence. This time it commonly takes the form of a participation in the intercourse of the parents via an identification with one of them. In the direct Oedipus complex it is via an identification with the parent of the same sex, and in the boy, for example, this is done by taking the place of the father and is symbolized by his murder. In the inverse complex the role taken is that of the parent of the opposite sex, leading to a homosexual coupling.

In order to indulge in such phantasies the facts of life have to be denied. Basically, these involve those facts which in reality are necessary to ensure a fertile creativity, and the process of perceiving this reality correctly involves the recognition of a couple from which the infant, by virtue of his size and immaturity, is excluded. Corollaries of this basic fact are the recognition of the difference between the sexes and between the generations. The infant has to argue that creative intercourse can take place just as well between a parent and a child or between a homosexual couple.

Again these issues are evaded when splitting is more total. The original split between the good and bad breast becomes complicated by the introduction of the father, who is also split into the good and bad penis. Two versions of the primal scene then coexist without contradiction, a loving one between the good mother and the good father and a hostile, often violent one, between the bad couple. As the splits lessen, perverse arguments have to be mounted to justify the phantasy that the parent prefers the child to an adult partner. In addition to the distinctions between generations and between sexes, a confusion between good and bad is maintained by perverse arguments. This confusion may lead to the creation of a terrifying combined object and it may be as a defence against this that further misrepresentations develop. Commonly these begin when the basic splits are reassembled, as Klein (1935) has pointed out, and Britton (1989) has reiterated, so that the good object is identified as the breast and the bad object as the penis.

Sometimes one or both parents play into these phantasies: for example, when the mother denigrates her husband in relation to her son, or when the father acts in ways which encourage him to be dismissed as insignificant. Such attitudes reinforce this kind of split and facilitate the removal of the father and his replacement by the child. In other cases, the split is between the good penis and the bad breast, and this leads to a turning to the father for protection from a persecuting mother. Again, it is when the splits lessen that the parents are seen as coming together and the 'supremely creative act' comes to be represented by the arrival of a sibling which threatens the omnipotence of the child.

Withdrawal to a narcissistic world where differences between the sexes and between the generations do not exist is once more offered as a refuge. Meltzer (1966), Chasseguet-Smirgel (1974, 1985), McDougall (1972), and Shengold (1988, 1989) have described these states in terms of the idealization of the anus and the creation of an anal world in which all differences are abolished. In this world everything is reduced to the same undifferentiated consistency, and it is important that the distinction between good and bad and hence between love and hate is also abolished. The individual then develops perverse relationships in which good objects are rejected and bad ones are idealized. This, as we have seen in Chapter 4, is characteristic of pathological organizations involving destructive narcissism, as Rosenfeld stressed.

The perverse solutions to these Oedipal facts of life are evident in the sexual perversions. The fact that a distinction between the sexes is essential to creative intercourse is denied by homosexuals, while that between the generations is ignored in paedophilia and child abuse. Sado-masochism is often turned to as integration leads to the possibility of a true recognition of painful reality. In sado-masochism love and hate are related in a perverse way and cruelty is indulged in without a full recognition of its damaging effects. Sado-masochistic phantasies give excitement and pleasure from cruelty which is not inhibited by a recognition of a hurt or damaged object. When splitting is active the damaged and the ideal objects are totally separated, but in perverse states an 'artful' statement links the two. The argument may be that women like to be hurt, or that if the child likes it, where is the harm? and so on. In the case of violent films and cartoons, sadism is often presented as harmless because the damaged object can be immediately resurrected and restored as new and the process of destruction and magical restoration can continue indefinitely. In other cruel situations the hurt is represented as a benefit such as those punishments which are done 'for the child's good'.

The third of Money-Kyrle's facts is 'the recognition of the inevitability of time and ultimately of death', and, as he suggests, this is of a different logical order from the first two facts. It is, one might say, a property of reality and one which affects the experience of all the facts of life. It is connected with the recognition of the fact that all good things have to come to an end, and it is precisely the fact that access to the breast cannot go on for ever that makes us aware of the reality of its existence in the external world. Similarly, it is the need for renewal and the reality of death which give rise to the recognition of the need for new life and creativity. The recognition of the reality of loss eventually leads to the need to confront our own mortality, and if this is not faced human values are distorted and perverted.

This fact of the reality of death is, of course, the central aspect of loss, and we have seen how in Freud's discussion of fetishism the patients he described had difficulty in acknowledging the death of their father. Distortions and misrepresentations of the reality of illness, ageing and death are connected with the difficulty of facing bad things as facts of life. Ugliness, violence, and evil are all associated with damage to and eventually with loss of our good objects and with the reality of our own mortality. These are some of the most difficult aspects of reality to face and their misrepresentation is often via the same perverse half-acceptance which Freud described. They are not usually classed as perversions but in my view it is useful to think of them as such. Misrepresentations here commonly lead to a romantic, sanitized world of idealizations in which good things go on for ever as in fairy-tales. In addition to narcissistic and sexual perversions, we could speak of romantic perversions of the reality of time. Stoller (1976) has suggested that this romantic defence is more prevalent among women, and represents a retreat into a dream world such as that created by romantic fiction. The male equivalent is pornographic masturbation, where the sexual element in the perversion is more explicit. The timelessness of the fantasy world is present in both.

Psychic retreats vary, as we have seen, both in their structure and in the anxiety they defend against. Some function predominantly as a retreat from paranoid-schizoid anxieties of fragmentation and persecution, while others are deployed primarily to deal with depressive affects such as guilt and despair. All, to varying degrees, serve as a retreat from reality, and in most, if not all, perverse mechanisms can be observed. Glover put forward the idea that perversion may protect the patient's reality sense and thus avoid psychotic manifestations (Glover 1933, 1964), and this might lead to the erroneous conclusion that perversion is rare in psychosis. Quite the contrary is true, and psychotic omnipotence is precisely what makes the enactment of perversion more likely and more dangerous. The error is similar to that which arose from Freud's statement that perversion is the negative of neurosis, which for a time led to the view that perversion was simply the expression of infantile sexuality and had no defensive function (see Gillespie 1964). Psychic retreats with a psychotic organization are no less likely to have perverse elements than the non-psychotic ones, and this arises because movements towards integration are far from absent in psychotic patients. These movements are particularly threatening to the psychotic patient, and when they occur they sometimes lead to a renewal of splitting and fragmentation but equally they sometimes lead to the creation of a psychotic organization which makes use of perverse mechanisms such as those described above (see Chapter 6).

A perverse relation to reality is consequently a feature of most, if not all, psychic retreats, and rather than present clinical material from a patient in whom this element is prominent I will review some of the patients discussed in previous chapters and try to illustrate the particular form of unreality seen in the retreat.

Clinical material

Mrs A (Chapter 2) withdrew to her bed where, for weeks on end, she did nothing but read novels. Her day-dreams involved journeys in the Sahara Desert which she idealized as a romantic place where life could be just sustained by careful rationing of water and provisions. In her sessions she withdrew into silence and would sometimes admit having fantasies of lying sun-bathing on a desert island, an image which was in keeping with the nonchalant, careless manner which she would adopt. The sadistic quality of this mood arose from the simultaneous awareness of the existence of an extremely needy patient who was longing for contact but was experienced as the responsibility of the analyst, and my efforts to reach her were simultaneously appreciated, mocked, or felt as a sadistic attack from a frustrated analyst.

From this retreat she would emerge and retreat again when hurt like a snail whose tentacles were touched. I discussed this feature in Chapter 2, when I described her dream of going out to get provisions and being shocked and also frightened by the girl who had been cut in two. Contact with me in that particular session was maintained until I raised the problem of an error in her cheque, and this led to an abrupt withdrawal.

After some progress she withdrew once more when she bruised her toe while working on the installing of central heating with her husband. She had failed to reach me because my phone was turned off and took to her bed and her novels, missing three sessions. When she returned, her material dealt with a memory of a room on the border where her family had stopped as they fled from her country of origin and where her mother was interrogated by the border guards. She also recalled that she stayed in a children's home for two weeks while her parents were said to have gone on holiday with her younger brother and where she remembered some wonderful dolls. Both places were undoubtedly associated with extreme anxiety, and both were idealized and formed part of the imagery of the psychic retreat. I thought these retreats, although awful in themselves, were seen as less horrible than the alternatives surrounding them, which in both situations were linked to the loss of her mother.

The awful dilemma of having to face reality which appears to be unbearable and is yet necessary for survival is solved by the creation of a retreat where reality is simultaneously accepted and denied. In her desert-island state of mind she was aware that she was neglected and deprived and at the same time comfortable and at ease.

Mr D (Chapter 7) formed alliances with powerful figures in the academic world in his attempt to keep his depression at bay. The organization he constructed helped him to engage in fantasies of a triumphant revenge while at the same time, by keeping these secret, he maintained a subservient and deferential attitude to his current employers and to his analyst. In fact, his hatred was expressed by the way in which he would ignore my interpretations and proceed to describe his excitement with new jobs and new girls which made me feel unimportant and helpless. While he seemed to recognize the effect this had on me, he denied his hatred and continued to maintain that he valued the analysis and that the problems which arose stemmed solely from his need to give his work priority which he was sure I understood. I was simultaneously a figure he valued and one he triumphed over, one he tried to preserve and one he tried to destroy. His manic state of mind was simultaneously an excited, triumphant state and one which damaged his objects and destroyed his prospects. These attitudes appeared to coexist without any contradiction becoming manifest.

Mr E's (Chapter 7) retreat was more masochistic, and involved a state of mind in which present suffering was tolerated and even idealized. In his dream, his gift of faeces was placed in an attractive box and treated simultaneously as a present and as an attack. He took a great deal of care and trouble over the analysis and at the same time had some awareness of the way in which his efforts blocked any analytic progress. In the psychic retreat he kept his objects in a state which was half alive and half dead and this meant that he was able neither to use them nor to relinquish them and mourn them. Occasionally, however, he was able to emerge from the retreat and to sustain a contact with the experience of loss which enabled a shift towards the depressive position to take place.

Mr C (Chapter 6) was more overtly psychotic and showed evidence of a mad retreat which threatened to break down. To compensate for and patch up a damaged ego he turned to omnipotent objects, Yahweh, neurologists, his analyst, with whom he wanted to identify and whose potency he sought. It was when he felt expelled from the retreat that he felt mad and tried to re-enter it by magical means, such as acquiring a prayer shawl. In the retreat he could do what he pleased, for example, shit where he wanted to because the disposal was the analyst's problem.

Despite the extent of the psychotic disintegration he had some insight into his damaged state when he said with a sense of loss that he once knew that 'I am I', meaning that he had once had a sense of identity and self. This enabled a transitory contact with the experience of loss which could not, however, be maintained. The perverse quality again arose from his awareness of this loss and his simultaneous denial of it as he resolved to solve his problems by omnipotence.

In this chapter the spatial representation of the retreat, as a desert island or as a room on the border, has been described, and I have tried to show how it is represented as an idealized haven and at the same time as a cruel place where life is only just sustainable. The perverse quality is associated with the coexistence of both these views.

At other times the retreat is represented not as a place but as a group of individuals bound together in an organization. The protection is provided by becoming a member of this group which comes to represent the safe haven. It is this second representation to which I refer when I speak of a pathological organization of the personality, and this has already been extensively discussed in previous chapters. In Chapter 9 I will emphasize this way of viewing retreats, and describe how perverse object relations play an important part in creating the rigidity and resistance to change of these structures.

Perverse relationships in pathological organizations[1]

The complex structure of pathological organizations of the personality has been discussed elsewhere in this book where I stressed the narcissistic nature of the object relationships involved. In this chapter I will describe how perverse relations between members of the organization, and with the self which is caught up in it, can contribute to the rigidity and stability of the organization.

When development occurs, whether in analysis or not, the patient feels stronger and more supported by his relationship with good objects so that he begins to have thoughts of escaping from the grip which the organization holds over him. He may make tentative movements outside the retreat, but he frequently returns once again as if convinced that he continues to depend on the organization for protection to avoid a catastrophe. In this way he remains stuck in the organization even though the conditions which led to his original dependence on it no longer exist and from other points of view he no longer seems to need it. The patient appears to be unable or unwilling to acknowledge that his circumstances have changed. Sometimes he is afraid to admit his improvement, since to do so is to stand up against an internal voice which tells him that the need for the organization still exists. This failure to admit improvement may appear as a kind of addiction to illness and to a dependence on the organization, and it is here that perverse elements become manifest and are revealed as binding the victim to the oppressor in ways which become very difficult to justify on grounds of need.

The internal situation is commonly presented by the patient as one where a healthy, sane, but weak part of the self is in the grip of a

---

1 This chapter is based on the paper entitled 'Perverse relationships between parts of the self: a clinical illustration' (Steiner 1982).

Mafia-like organization which he is powerless to resist. I believe this is misleading, and I will try to show that a perverse relationship exists and that the so-called 'healthy but weak' part of the self colludes and knowingly allows itself to be taken over by the narcissistic gang. Perverse relationships between members of the organization bind them to one another and often to a leader, in ways which ensure loyalty. These very same perverse links enmesh and imprison the dependent parts of the self which cannot remain outside the organization even when there is a disapproval of its methods and discomfort about benefiting from its advantages.

Perhaps equally important is the way the analyst is drawn into the organization. He too is unable to stay aloof and uncorrupted by perverse seduction and intimidation. The situation often corresponds to the struggle of a child in a perverse family where both the patient and the analyst participate and where the basic structure is made rigid by the roles which each of the parties are obliged to enact. Within this rigidity roles are sometimes interchangeable, and the patient sometimes sees himself as a victim and sometimes as a persecutor and the analyst may find himself placed in the complementary role.

The perverse quality of this type of relationship has been observed by a number of authors. Joseph (1975), while studying patients who are 'difficult to reach', stressed the tricky way in which they can twist and manipulate the analyst. Although mainly concerned with problems of technique, she describes a pseudo-cooperative part of the self which is actively keeping another, more needy and potentially responsive part split off. At other times a split-off part of the self appears to watch and destructively prevent any real contact from being made. Joseph makes it clear that if the situation in the transference is examined in detail it can be understood not simply as a global defence but in terms of complex and highly organized facets of the patient's personality. She shows the subtle nature of the acting out in the transference, and emphasizes the pressure on the analyst to collude and allow himself to be manipulated into taking a role where he acts out a part of the patient's self rather than analyses it. Several writers (Sandler 1976; Sandler and Sandler 1978; Rosenfeld 1978; Langs 1978) describe the way the analyst's own blind spots contribute to the tendency to engage in collusive acting out. Rosenfeld (1971a) suggests that pathological fusions of the instincts produce a state in which, instead of neutralizing the destructive impulses, the admixture of libido may actually make it even more dangerous. This implies a perverse interaction between parts of the self, and Grotstein (1979) appears to have something similar in mind when he refers to 'collusive symbiosis' between a psychotic and a neurotic personality organization resulting in what he calls a 'perverse amalgam'.

A complex situation develops which may be difficult to unravel but which can usually be recognized as the analyst becomes familiar with the patient's world and how it operates. The basic structure of the organization, as we have seen, is represented as a group, gang, or network of objects in a relationship. This organization originates in the nuclear family and begins with the Oedipal trio, but extends to the wider family and from them to other objects in the patient's surroundings. Each of the objects in the inner world has parts of the self projected into them, and this contributes to their complexity and to their rigidity. These objects are often chosen because they are suitable for the containment of particular parts of the self. In this way dependent elements in the self tend to be projected into one group of objects and destructive parts of the self are projected into other figures which may themselves be chosen for their power, cruelty, or ruthlessness. The dependent elements are then trapped in a sado–masochistic relationship with the powerful, aggressive elements and the patient may locate himself in one or other group or alternately may feel himself to be a helpless observer rather than a participant. At the same time he cannot free himself because to leave would be to abandon elements of himself which he has projected. Moreover, because he is simultaneously identified with both victim and oppressor, he fears that to leave the organization would bring onto himself a violent attack.

Each of the members of the network or gang remains insecure and even if he feels he is temporarily in favour he knows that the tables can be turned and that he may find himself a victim. Each member identifies with both victim and oppressor, and each is held in the same type of perverse grip. The grip gains its power from seduction and collusion on the one hand and from threats of violence on the other.

These perverse links can be recognized to operate in various degrees in most pathological organizations, and it is possible to review the cases discussed in previous chapters from this point of view. Rather than do this, however, in this chapter I will present clinical material which offers further illustration of an organization with such perverse relationships.

Clinical material

The patient (Mr F) was a 40-year-old doctor who sought analysis after a period of anxiety, confusion, and depersonalization. Although reasonably successful professionally, he felt obliged to give up clinical work for research and was painfully aware that he led a restricted life, unable to maintain personal relationships.

His parents were well-meaning, devout people, very involved with the church and with high expectations for their children. His father was depressed for a time when the patient was a small child and remained disappointed with his own professional achievements. His mother was very rarely mentioned, and remained a shadowy figure who seemed preoccupied with the patient's younger sister and appeared to hand over some of the care of the patient to the father. His older brother had to some extent rebelled against the family's expectations and did labouring jobs in order to find himself as a painter, at which he achieved some success. The patient's sister, younger by 18 months, was a source of great jealousy mostly unacknowledged by the patient. Both siblings were married with children, and the patient felt, by comparison, that he was defective.

He was a tall, very thin, awkward but attractive-looking man who set great store on health and sometimes jogged to his session. A striking feature was that his anxiety, while quite evident as he came into the room, would disappear as he gave me a formal nod of greeting and lay down. It seemed as though the couch represented a haven where he could feel protected from anxiety, and later in the analysis this experience was linked to his difficulty in getting up out of bed at home. If he had anything difficult to face at school or in his relationships he would try to stay in bed and even became ill with anxiety. Often his mother appeared to collude by insisting that he stay in bed. Although apparently free of anxiety and talking in a superior way which appeared to give him much pleasure, he also conveyed an experience of great suffering. He often referred to the way life was passing him by and to his fear that unless I could help him to emerge from his present state his life would never have any meaning for him. Very occasionally he did let me see a needy, dependent part of himself – for example, when he described with feeling how as a small boy he forgot to get off the bus near his home and had to walk up a steep hill alone and miserable. Mostly, however, his dependent needs could only be hinted at in part, it seemed, because of a great fear of being mocked.

Sometimes, especially at the beginning of sessions, his feelings came through more clearly. Once, for example, he was horrified to find that a sticky substance had got onto his hand from the door handle, and this affected him in a way which allowed a direct expression of his horror and disgust of bodily secretions. He had refused milk and eggs since early childhood and usually also avoided meat, living largely on health foods, which he considered a superior form of nourishment.

It was possible to identify a narcissistic organization in which destructive parts of the self and destructive objects were idealized, which partly gained its strength from an identification with what the patient called 'top-brass' people and which appeared to gain a hold on the personality by presenting itself as a suitable guardian for the dependent, needy self. In fact, the superior way of talking served to undermine the value of anything I might say and the narcissistic organization kept the libidinal self stunted and underdeveloped by preventing anything alive, colourful, and nourishing from entering his life.

The chief point I want to make via the clinical material is that the patient developed considerable insight into the fact that he was dominated by a destructive, sadistic organization which prevented his growth and that, despite this insight, he continued to collude with the organization in a perverse way. As a subsidiary theme, I want to suggest that a clarification of the situation was made more difficult by the fact that we were not dealing with a simple split between good and bad. Instead, both the needy and the protective parts of his personality were complex, each containing some good and some bad elements. This fact disguised the essentially destructive nature of the protective organization and justified a collusion with it by the dependent parts of the self.

About 15 months after the beginning of the analysis he described how one of his many exciting platonic relationships had come to an end when the girl in question told him she had another man.

He then reported a dream in which he broke into her flat, knowing where the key was kept, and got into her bed while she was out. When she returned with her boy-friend, he called out to warn her of his presence and the boy-friend walked into the bedroom. The dream ended as he realized that he would soon be asked to leave.

When I interpreted in terms of a small boy with a desire for warmth and comfort who wanted to get close to me, he replied that he had no real desire for the girl. I then suggested that although he now denied this desire, in his dream he was persuaded to get into the bed by a part of him that claimed to look after him and tempted him with warmth and comfort. However, all the time he knew very well what the outcome would be and that perhaps he was right and that his real desire was for humiliation and cruelty.

I thought there was a part of him in touch with his needs, and therefore susceptible to this persuasion, but that this part was dominated by a search for cruelty, and that he set up situations where he was bound to be humiliated and thrown out. I think he wanted the essential cruelty of the dream to be repeated in the session and was nudging me to interpret in a rejecting way, emphasizing his intrusiveness and voyeurism.

In my view, the needy, dependent part of the self had been seduced and was now colluding with a narcissistic organization which promised to look after him but in fact was dominated by sadistic motives. His insight, derived from many repetitions of this type of outcome, did not lead to any change because the libidinal self had by now been perverted and got gratification of a masochistic kind.

Another dream illustrates the complex nature of the object relationships in his inner world.

He was going on a journey and the little trolley under his suitcase rolled into the road and was bent in a collision with traffic. Next, he was at a railway station with a great deal of luggage. He was so impatient he decided to get on the next train wherever it went, saying to himself that anyway they all went in the same direction, but he couldn't get all his luggage onto the platform and left some behind, in particular his mother's cello.

His associations were that this cello had recently been damaged and ought to be repaired. When this had happened he had bought himself a new fibreglass case for his own cello which, however, he had never played and in fact had lent to a friend. He wondered if he could even take it up again.

I thought he was in touch with depressive feelings as he struggled with his baggage which represented his internal objects. Some of these were damaged and they were too much for him to cope with, even though he recognized them as his responsibility. Reparation was not possible because his own creativity represented by the trolley was bent. He had an operation at the age of 12 to repair an undescended testicle which until then had escaped notice, and this left him with grave doubts about his masculinity.

In this state he was particularly susceptible to the seductions and persuasions of the narcissistic part of himself. Against all reason he was persuaded to believe that any train would do, just as he believed that any girl would do to gratify his perverse sexuality. The libidinal self capable of growth and insight seemed to be represented by his own cello which, probably because of his extreme sensitivity, was protected by its fibreglass case or by being given to a friend for safe-keeping. It was therefore not available for use at the time when he needed it, and this made it even more difficult to resist the narcissistic persuasion.

Later he was able to tell me that he had actually once left some luggage behind at a station, at a time when he was very anxious. He had stayed on one holiday at medical school to finish a research project, and with almost everyone else gone he felt desperately alone. However, he sustained himself with excitement over his project, which, like so many others, he thought was brilliant until his excitement collapsed. He was able to describe to me then how he became miserable and frightened and feared he was going mad. For a time after this session he was able to stay more in touch and to acknowledge worries about himself. The shift seemed to be connected with the fact that I was able to avoid collusion with a superior part of him so that he did not experience me as either denying or looking down on his sense of inadequacy.

In another dream he was a tourist in Nepal and was shown a boy who had swollen eyes and was weeping. A Nepalese doctor was called but the treatment consisted of putting the boy out of his misery. The boy was asked if he wanted to die and he said that he did, so the doctor began to attack him with blows on his head, and when this failed he began to saw through the neck in a very painful way. The patient wondered why as a tourist he was watching all this and he felt quite powerless to intervene, but was unable to stop himself watching. He was reminded of a film in which an American had to watch his Chinese friend being tortured and decided to shoot him as an act of mercy.

This material seemed to demonstrate how imprisoned he was by a cruel, destructive part of himself which professed to be his friend. If he admitted he was an ill, weeping boy he was convinced I would collude with his cruelty and that he would receive Nepalese medicine of the kind shown by the doctor in the dream. On the other hand, if he turned to me as a helpful analyst and allowed me to befriend him as the American had done in the film, he believed that the narcissistic organization threatened him with torture. At the same time he was fascinated by the cruelty and got a voyeuristic gratification from watching it. Contact with his dependent needs was felt to be so painful and humiliating that he experienced the analysis as a cruelty which nevertheless he agreed to by coming to his session each day.

He began another session by handing me a cheque, saying that this time he had already torn it out of the cheque book. He referred to it as his 'monthly ritual' and went on, as he often did, with what he called a 'weedy' joke. A defeated Chinese general was told by an English general that the secret of success was prayer. 'But we pray too,' said the Chinese, and the Englishman replied that perhaps God did not understand Chinese!

He was reminded of this joke by a dream in which a Chinese was giving him a Nazi hat.

He had been thinking that the German army was really very different from the SS: the army may shoot people but the SS tortures them.

The monthly ritual referred to earlier work in which tearing out the cheque was associated with the operation on his testicle, leaving him 'in the same boat as women', and which he felt he was forced to accept without protest. In the session he felt like a weedy infant unable to fight back as the normal German army might and unable to protest or to communicate his feelings because he felt that, like his parents, I would not understand his infantile language. In the circumstance he was easily persuaded that accepting the Nazi hat was justified. It seemed to represent the way he suppressed all conscious protest, converting it instead into a secret, perverse cruelty tormenting himself and me.

A few days later he came in wet and miserable, having jogged to his session in bad weather. He said he was relieved that he had decided to lie down even though it might wet the pillow.

Next he described a dream in which he attended a private view of a film about the Chinese book of prophecy, the I-Ching (he pronounced this as Eee Ching). A woman was present with a yellow and black striped dress like a wasp. Then he was sitting in a bath peeling carrots and potatoes. Two 'wet' missionaries were present, 'Wet in Mrs Thatcher's sense', he added.[1]

He remembered how, once while he was on duty, two missionaries had come to the hospital seeking treatment and that he had sent them away.

I suggested that there was something sad and also perhaps comic about the picture of himself in the bath which I thought might be connected with an examination of his genitals which he used to do in the bath, and which led to the discovery that he only had one testicle. I wondered if it wasn't one of his 'weedy' jokes, and that perhaps the missionaries represented the analysis and that when, as today, he felt especially wet, miserable, and weedy he projected this onto me and sent me away.

He seemed affected by this interpretation and after thinking for a while elaborated on the *I-Ching*, saying that he had been introduced to it by a friend called Prue, who played a large part in his fantasies, and he mentioned the name Prue several times. I asked if he connected this with the medical word for itching, which I linked with his way of pronouncing *I-Ching*. He agreed, and said that this gave him a shock memory. Recently a friend accused him of prurience and he had looked up the word and found it connected with itching. I suggested that he was reluctant to admit a prurient interest in my state of mind if he saw me as 'wet' in Mrs Thatcher's sense, but that he was also expressing a fear that my interest in him would be prurient, and that I would not understand how he felt when he came so wet and miserable and aware that there were things wrong with him. He returned to the

---

1 At that time the Prime Minister had called 'wet' those members of her cabinet she considered to be weak.

110

dream in the next session via an association to the wasp-like woman. He recalled seeing a film called *The Sting* in which a policeman pretended to be enjoying a joke and suddenly became violent.

Although he wanted the analysis to deal with his worries, such as those about his genitals, it was easier to turn the experience into a weedy joke which allowed him to project the misery and to get excited by his cleverness. When he did so he was terrified of being caught out and of humiliation and cruelty. Nevertheless, he could not resist the temptation to free himself of his feelings of need and dependence even though his experience showed him repeatedly how each such enactment ended in disaster.

The patient's distinction between the German army and the SS represented for him the differentiation between two parts of his personality. That associated with the SS was based on an omnipotent grandiosity, and functioned by projecting and imprisoning the needy self in his analyst and then cruelly mocking and tormenting both himself and me. He was at the mercy of a narcissistic organization whose cruelty and ruthlessness was to some extent contained by a more reality-based part of him which was able to function in a reasonable and logical way.

The self-destructiveness which could be recognized without difficulty both in analysis and in his everyday life was hidden from himself by being disguised and idealized. He could not ignore the libidinal, needy side of him and he knew how awful it was to be a small, lost boy feeling wet and humiliated by his dependence on his objects. Because he could not get rid of these feelings completely he had to establish a perverse liaison in which the needy child agreed to be humiliated. Only rarely was this part of him able to protest directly at the frustration he had to endure. At those times when he did get in touch with his needs and was able to protest he felt aggressive but not perverse – namely, more like the German army than the SS – but such protest was made more dangerous by the fact that the narcissistic structure was then projected into the analyst and he believed that he would be treated cruelly rather than understood. To protest would be to acknowledge his separateness and to stand up against the organization, which he feared to do.

If, as often happened, I failed to stay sufficiently in touch to make him feel understood, he was particularly likely to be drawn into a collusion with the narcissistic organization. This was especially true when I could not resist clever, witty interactions with him which I think he experienced as my abandoning his real needs to collude in a perverse way and gratify *my* narcissism. Even when I avoided this, however, he often felt that I only did so by trying hard, and he thought

I had to exert a great effort not to laugh at his jokes. The cruelty he expected was like that of the wasp woman, and seemed to correspond to a fear of perversion and prurience. He saw his objects as damaged like his mother's cello or bent like the trolley in his dream. The part of himself more associated with a non-perverse protest was too afraid of an open conflict and turned instead to collusion with the cruel, secret spoiling and devaluing of the analytic work.

One of the features I want to stress is that the patient had insight of a kind into the mechanisms I have been describing. He knew that his superior devaluing of things he actually admired was stunting his development, and he seemed to know that he was allowing this to happen. In his dreams an ill boy would be persuaded to allow himself to be tortured, and in the sessions he knew that he could protest and enlist my aid when he felt something too cruel was going on. Occasionally, he saw that constructive work was possible and there was a general feeling of appreciation of his analysis. Nevertheless, he could not resist attacking it and getting masochistic gratification from the excited attempts at destruction.

Just as constructive elements become attached to the narcissistic part of the self, so can perverse elements be located in the libidinal part of the personality. I believe that this situation arises when splitting breaks down and good is not properly separated from bad. In Chapter 3 I described how a breakdown of splitting can lead to confusional states such as those described by Rosenfeld (1950) and Klein (1957). If such confusional states cannot be resolved by further idealization and splitting, fragmentation results and the fragments become re-assembled in an artificial way to produce a pathological organization of the personality. Destructive elements of the self in association with destructive objects are personified and projected into objects which are then organized by a leader into a narcissistic gang. The dependent, needy part of the self is then imprisoned by the gang and is helpless to escape or to alter the situation. This is how the patient presents the state of affairs, sometimes consciously and sometimes emerging as an interpretation of unconscious phantasy.

I believe it is possible to see that this type of relationship between victim and persecutor does not in fact result from a split but from an artificial and contrived partition between good and bad. On closer inspection many good elements are discernible in the narcissistic organization, which does attempt to protect and look after the child but fails to master the cruelty. And, perhaps more important, perverse elements are to be found in the needy, dependent self which often asks for and accepts the perverse protection and exploitation despite insight into what is going on.

Normal splitting can be thought of as a cleavage along natural lines of fissure as occurs when a piece of marble or granite is split when struck with a hammer. Pathological conglomeration of the kind I am describing is then more of an artificial division, like a piece of salami being sliced by a knife. Good and bad parts of the self, like pieces of meat and fat in the salami, are to be found on both sides and adhere to each other in a sticky way. The glue which binds elements of a pathological organization together is perversion, and because of the gratification which this provides both to victim and to perpetrator it is very difficult to give up.

The following material shows how the organization can function as a defence against confusion. The patient regularly brought his daily newspaper with him to the session, and one day, while discussing this, he described a ritual which took place each Saturday when he bought a paper and then took his washing to the laundrette for a service wash.

He then described a dream in which he was occupying a small, dark room in a holiday cottage with his mother and several others, perhaps with their mothers. It was dark and gloomy and he wanted to find a way out. When he got outside he saw a lot of Russian soldiers, and he explained that this was not an occupation force because they had been invited in by the government somehow in connection with the fact that the Russians had invaded Bulgaria. Then he saw some British soldiers but thought they looked rather disorderly, walking and chatting rather than goose-stepping.

His associations were to the previous evening when he had visited friends who had spoken about the cottage they share with their parents, and he had watched his friend take the washing out of the machine. He noticed that children's clothes, the husband's clothes, and the wife's underwear were all mixed up together and he thought the underwear looked tatty and worn. I interpreted that, in his sessions, he felt he brought parts of himself to be cleaned up and sorted out and he waited for me to do the work in the manner of a service wash. He projected parts of himself into me and then felt trapped and very confused, not being sure if he felt himself to be a child, a man, or a woman. To escape from this confusion he turned to the newspaper, at that time full of accounts of Soviet invasions. Although he described British troops, in his dream they were rather tatty, like the underwear, and he felt he had to invite the Russian troops in to sort out the confusion.

He went on to say that an invading army might liberate a country and lead it to prosper as West Germany had done. I was aware that it would be difficult to sort this out because there was no clear differentiation between a liberating army which might allow him to prosper and a totalitarian occupying force which was invited in to make order out

113

of confusion. I interpreted that just as he felt he invaded my mind with all his dirty washing, so he feared my thoughts would invade his mind, and he was not sure if the invasion would imprison him or help to free him from a totalitarian part of himself which he turns to when confused.

He then described how he had arranged for a girl to share his flat for a while, and that she would clean and decorate in lieu of rent. He was obviously interested in this girl and was told that she had a fiancé in Bulgaria who could not get out to join her. I interpreted that he was bringing another factor behind his ambivalence. Although he was generally against totalitarian ways of thinking, the Russian regime could serve not only to keep order but to give expression to his envy and jealousy. He could prevent the couple coming together and thus ensure that he would continue to be looked after. He colluded with the narcissistic organization to escape from a confusional state and was then the passive collaborator in an envious invasion. His contempt for the tatty underwear and the more humane British army thinly concealed his envy of the family he found so desirable and felt left out of.

Conclusions

In this chapter I have presented clinical material which emphasized the way a narcissistic part of the personality can acquire a disproportionate power by gaining a hold on the healthier parts of the personality, and I have suggested that it does this to the extent that it can persuade these parts to enter into perverse liaisons. An understanding of these liaisons can help the analyst to resist some of the pressure to act out with his patient.

In this material it is possible to recognize how the patient dealt with his feelings of being small and dependent. By turning to powerful figures, his 'top-brass' people, he got rid of these uncomfortable feelings and was able to project them and then mistreat them in himself and in others. At the same time he opposed these cruel methods and had some insight into the way the 'top-brass' let him down. Nevertheless, he was always persuaded that, 'this time it might be different'. In addition to such seductive persuasion, he was clearly fascinated by sadism and ruthlessness which entered into his dreams and fantasies and held him enthralled. He was often obliged to watch cruelty and was powerless to intervene and unable to tear himself away.

The existence of such perverse attractions may keep the patient addicted to defensive manoeuvres beyond the point when they serve any adaptive function. They also contribute to the patient's despair, because he recognizes the strength of the hold they have on him. He cannot then believe that he would be able to resist the pull even if he has insight into the self-destructive nature of the addiction. This is one of the factors which makes the patient feel that the whole organization has to be destroyed before he can be free of it, and such omnipotent motives may also be induced in the analyst.

I have tried to show that we are dealing here not with a split between good and bad, but with the consequences of a breakdown in splitting and a reassembling of the fragments into a complex mixture under the dominance of an omnipotent narcissistic structure. In order to free the healthy, sane part of the patient, we have to understand the whole situation. I believe this includes the propensity of the patient to present himself, both to himself and to the analyst, as the innocent victim. We have to recognize the sense of helplessness, but also those occasions when a collusion develops and the patient gets a perverse gratification from the domination of the narcissistic organization. Insight into the domination may then not be enough, and the collusion has also to be exposed. If this can be achieved, the patient can sometimes come to accept the existence of a part of himself as truly destructive, which he has to learn to live with, which can be contained and may be modified, but which cannot be disowned.

10

Two types of pathological organization in *Oedipus the King* and *Oedipus at Colonus*[1]

In this chapter I will turn to literature rather than the consulting room for my material and will discuss the way Oedipus is presented as grappling with reality and self-knowledge in the two plays about him by Sophocles. In the first play, *Oedipus the King*, I believe we can recognize that Oedipus both knew and did not know the truth of what he was doing. I will argue that he knew but *turned a blind eye* to the knowledge, and that this left him in a retreat where his relation with reality was perverse. In *Oedipus at Colonus*, in which Sophocles shows Oedipus as a blind old man facing death, we see a very different person, this time dealing with reality in a more drastic way, by a *retreat from truth to omnipotence*. A marked change can be seen in the character of Oedipus in the two plays, and I believe this change occurs when Oedipus blinds himself and as a result finds himself in a situation analogous to the psychotic who attacks his own perceptual apparatus. In both plays Oedipus is presented as having to evade reality, but the two methods employed are very different and reflect the operation of two different types of pathological organization of the personality.[2]

These views are a significant departure from the usual interpretation of the plays, in which Oedipus is seen as an innocent man struggling with relentless fate, and they are largely based on the work of Philip Vellacott, an idiosyncratic classicist, who is known for his translations of Aeschylus and Euripides (Vellacott 1956, 1961, 1971) but whose book on *Oedipus the King* (Vellacott 1971) has been either attacked or dismissed by most critics. Although there are several aspects of

---

1 This chapter is based on two earlier papers: 'Turning a blind eye' (Steiner 1985), and 'The retreat from truth to omnipotence in *Oedipus at Colonus*' (Steiner 1990b).

2 *Antigone*, the third play on the Theban theme, is also relevant to many of the issues touched on here but would take us too far afield to be discussed in the present chapter.

Vellacott's argument with which I disagree, I found his basic approach extremely convincing and enlightening to me as a psychoanalyst.

There are, of course, many commentaries on the plays of Sophocles, and over 300 psychoanalytic papers on the Oedipus myth (Edmunds and Ingber 1977), which I will not attempt to review. A study by Rudnytsky (1987) covers a wide field and looks not only at the plays but also at the way they influenced Freud. Winnington-Ingram's (1980) book can serve as a good example of the writings of a Greek scholar who accepts the classical view that Oedipus had no knowledge of who it was he killed or who it was he married. Moreover, like most scholars, he argues that, in Colonus, Oedipus is finally able to gain recognition of the wrongs done to him and acquire heroic stature through his suffering. His denial of guilt is then fitting to his status as he faces death.

It is important to note that the new approach to the plays is by no means intended to replace the classical view which makes up the manifest content of the plays. Like the manifest content of a dream, however, I believe it is possible to see various layers of unconscious and half-conscious meaning which exist alongside it, and which give depth to the meaning of the plays and help us to understand the profound effect they have on us.

The story of Oedipus the King

The tragedy of Oedipus begins when Laius, King of Thebes, is told by the Oracle of Apollo that his fate is to die at the hand of his son. In order to avoid this prophecy, Laius and his wife Jocasta pierce the feet of the new-born baby and give him to a shepherd to be left to die in the neighbouring mountains of Cithaeron. The shepherd takes pity on the child, and saves his life so that Oedipus finds himself brought up in the royal court of Corinth as the son of the childless King Polybus and his Queen Merope. As a young man, he attends a banquet where someone drinks too much and suggests he is not the true son of his parents. Oedipus, not satisfied by their reassurance, goes to seek the truth from the Oracle at Delphi.

The Oracle is evasive over the question of his origins, but instead repeats the prophecy made earlier to Laius, and warns Oedipus that he is fated to kill his father and marry his mother. In order to avoid this fate and to preserve Polybus and Merope, he decides never to return to Corinth, and setting off in the opposite direction he comes to a place where three roads meet, and there confronts a carriage preceded by a herald, who pushes him out of the way. In anger he hits back, and when the occupant of the carriage strikes him, he retaliates by killing the man and his four servants; one man only escapes to take the news back to Thebes. Oedipus continues on his way and, arriving at Thebes, he finds the city tyrannized by the Sphinx, who strangles all those who fail to guess her riddle.

The riddle goes as follows: 'There is on earth a thing two footed and four footed and three footed which has one voice . . . but when it goes on most feet then its speed is feeblest.' Oedipus accepts the challenge and solves the riddle, perhaps helped by the fact that the word for 'two footed' is *di-pous* while his own name, 'Oedipus', means swollen feet, and refers to the injury inflicted by his parents. The answer he gave was that a man crawls on four feet as an infant, walks on two as an adult, and hobbles with the help of a stick in old age. The defeated Sphinx commits suicide and the grateful city offers Oedipus the recently vacated crown of Thebes and the recently widowed Jocasta as Queen.

Oedipus rules Thebes for some seventeen years until the city is once more afflicted with disaster in the form of a plague, and once more the oracle is consulted. This is the point at which Sophocles' *Oedipus* begins. It opens with the people pleading with Oedipus to help them in their suffering from the plague. Jocasta's brother, Creon, interrupts them with the long–awaited message from the Oracle which states that the city is polluted by the continuing presence of the murderer of Laius. Oedipus swears to find and banish the wrongdoer, and the ancient soothsayer Tiresias is sent for to identify the guilty man. This he at first refuses to do, but when Oedipus becomes childishly abusive, Tiresias gets angry and tells him in plain terms first that he, Oedipus, is the killer of Laius and next, by clear implication, that he is not the son of Polybus and Merope as he claims, but of Jocasta and Laius. It is he, therefore, who is 'the unholy polluter of the land . . . living in shameful intercourse with his nearest of kin'.[1]

To these accusations Oedipus replies with more abuse, and begins to accuse Creon of plotting to overthrow him. Jocasta enters and Oedipus heeds her appeal and becomes more reasonable. When she discovers that he is accused by Tiresias of killing Laius, she reassures him that prophets are not to be trusted as was clear in the prophecy given to Laius, which she explains was evidently false because first, Laius' son was exposed and left to die, and secondly, Laius was killed by bandits at a place where three roads met. Oedipus is disturbed and begins to question Jocasta about the details of the King's death. How was he attended? What did he look like? Who brought the news back to Thebes? Then, explaining his forebodings, he gives an account of his

---

1 The quotations from *The Theban Plays* are taken from the translation by E.F. Watling (1947).

origins in Corinth, his doubts about his parentage, his message from the Oracle, and finally a description of the slaying of the man at the place where three roads meet. If the man he killed was Laius, he is doomed. The witness at the time, however, stated that Laius was killed by a band of robbers, and although the evidence pointing to Oedipus seems inescapable, there is just a chance that the witness will stick to his story of robbers and everyone agrees to suspend judgement until they have interrogated him. The issue of Oedipus' parents is also ignored, despite Jocasta's account of the prophecy given to Laius, Oedipus' account of that given to him, and the unspoken evidence known to Oedipus and surely to Jocasta of the scars on his feet.

These are only brought into the open with the arrival of the shepherd from Corinth who announces the death of Polybus. Oedipus and Jocasta rejoice at this news as if it should be a source of reassurance, proving again the falseness of prophecies. Oedipus then raises the absurdly remote danger that he may still inadvertently marry the aged Queen of Corinth, and Jocasta repeatedly tries to reassure him. The Corinthian shepherd, apparently amazed that they know so little of the truth, explains his parentage to Oedipus, having himself been the man who handed over the baby to Polybus. Finally, the Theban shepherd who witnessed the killing of Laius appears, and proves to be the same servant who saved Oedipus as a baby.

Jocasta now realizes the whole truth and, becoming increasingly distraught, pleads with Oedipus not to pursue the matter further. Oedipus, however, continues with the denial and even introduces a new argument. If he is not the son of Polybus, he is possibly not royal at all, probably the son of a slave girl, and that is why Jocasta is making such a fuss. Jocasta rushes out, and under the threat of torture the shepherd tells the whole story. The mood changes and Oedipus gives up the denial and prevarication to face the truth and acknowledge his guilt. This is a truly heroic moment which in my view forms the climax of the play. It is followed by a description from a messenger of events which take place out of sight within the palace. Oedipus finds Jocasta has hanged herself and, taking her brooches, he blinds himself with them. The play ends with Creon in control and Oedipus expecting to be banished.[1]

Vellacott's interpretation

Vellacott's detailed analysis of *Oedipus the King* (1971) put forward the

---

1 The section of the play which describes Oedipus facing his guilt and the subsequent catastrophe are so important that I discuss them further later in the chapter.

heretical idea that, far from being ignorant and hence innocent of what he did, Oedipus, and others also, knew that he had killed King Laius and married his widow. Vellacott also shows that if Oedipus had followed up all the indications which cast doubt on his parentage, he would have discovered that he was the son of Laius and Jocasta and he would have at that point recognized the crimes of parricide and incest which were to be revealed so tragically at the climax of the play. It seems to me less certain that he fully knew all these facts, and it is more plausible that he half-knew them, and decided to turn a blind eye to this half-knowledge. His ignorance was made possible by the fact that neither he, nor Creon, Jocasta or the Elders of Thebes, chose to pursue enquiries, and this arose from their reluctance to know the truth. Instead, they dealt with unwelcome reality by *turning a blind eye*.

The contrasting classical view, which is generally accepted, is that Oedipus acted without conscious knowledge and was therefore innocent. Because of what he did he became a polluted man, looked on with horror and pity, but he had no reason to feel guilt. Vellacott's careful reading of the text suggests that Sophocles put forward both views simultaneously, and this interpretation allows us to link the situation he describes with the state of mind we encounter in our patients, where something can be both known and not known.[1]

Once we are alerted to the possibility, it is easy to see that Oedipus must have realized that he had killed Laius and married his widow. He arrived in Thebes having just killed a man who was evidently important because he had a herald and retinue and must have found the city buzzing with the news of the death of the King. It is true that both he and everyone else was preoccupied with the threat of the Sphinx, but it is impossible to think that he did not connect these events. He solved the riddle of the Sphinx and accepted the hand of Jocasta without qualm because, as André Green has suggested (Green 1987), the desire to enjoy Laius's throne and Jocasta's bed made him a poor logician.

Later he asks why there was no enquiry into Laius' death, but neither Creon, nor Jocasta nor the Elders wanted to know. They for their individual reasons preferred to accept the new King and to welcome the overthrow of the Sphinx without asking awkward questions. Later we learn that Tiresias knew and kept the knowledge to himself for

---

1 Vellacott in fact suggests that Sophocles had two audiences in mind, the ordinary one who would respond to the classical view, and a few elite individuals who could see beyond this to the revised view Vellacott is putting. I feel this weakens his argument, because one aspect of the play's greatness is the way it touches depths in all of us and it is surely much truer to say that each of us responds in both ways, like Oedipus, accepting that we know and do not know simultaneously.

seventeen years, and then he argues that it is better not to speak because, 'When wisdom brings no profit, to be wise is to suffer'. It seems to me clear that not only did all the chief characters turn a blind eye but that an unconscious or half-conscious collusion took place, since if any one of them had exercised their curiosity the truth would easily have come out.[1]

Did Oedipus also realize that Laius was his father and Jocasta his mother? This was perhaps not so obvious, and yet the play is riddled with hints that could and should have been followed up. In order to maintain that he is the son of Polybus and Merope, Oedipus turns a blind eye to the fact that he went to consult the Oracle precisely because he had doubts over his parentage which the Oracle did nothing to allay. With the prophecy ringing in his ears he kills a man old enough to be his father and marries a woman old enough to be his mother. He turns a blind eye, as does Jocasta, to the scars on his feet which he speaks of as a stigma carried from the cradle which gave him his name.

What is even more remarkable is how in the course of the play itself both the characters on the stage and we in the audience are persuaded by the skill of the dramatist to turn a blind eye as the truth is put before us. Thus in the first five minutes of the play Tiresias asserts without any possibility of being misunderstood that Oedipus himself is the cursed polluter of Thebes, that he is living in sinful union with the one he loves, and that he does not realize whose son he is. He tells him that he has sinned against his own, on earth and in the grave, and finally that his mother's and father's curse will sweep him out of the city. Oedipus dismisses this as a plot to discredit him and reacts with abuse and counter-accusations, but the Elders, immediately after hearing these clear pronouncements from someone they respect second only to Apollo himself, start to sing of 'The shedder of blood, the doer of deeds unnamed', and ask, 'Who is this man, where is he? In forest or cave, a wild ox roaming the mountains.' They clearly do not want to make the connection, and neither do we in the audience as we watch out the drama. We know the truth but turn a blind eye to it as we identify with the characters we are watching.

Oedipus is able to keep his guilty secret hidden, perhaps in some measure from himself as well as from others, and to rule Thebes until a second plague, this time attacking anything to do with procreation, demands that the truth be sought out. Up to this point we have had the cover-up of truth and now the time for exposing this cover-up has come. I discovered an unusual theatre director who put it this way:

---

1 Stewart (1961) has discussed Jocasta's complicity from a slightly different point of view.

My dear, I am sorry to say this, but no one has understood before now that *Oedipus* is not about the revelation of truth but about the cover-up of truth. Everybody knows who Oedipus is from the start and everybody is covering up. Just like Watergate. Just like all through history – the lie is what societies are based upon.

(Pilikian 1974)

In fact, however, when he is forced to face reality and can maintain the cover-up no longer, Oedipus does so with great courage. It is not easy for him, and we see him vacillating and struggling with his ambivalence, but this only makes his final achievement the more impressive. I will argue that this movement towards truth is tragically reversed in *Oedipus at Colonus*, and for this eccentric view of the play I am also indebted to Philip Vellacott. I believe that this reversal actually begins in the first play at the point when Oedipus blinds himself, and before elaborating Vellacott's view of Colonus, I will look again at the climax of *Oedipus the King*. Here it seems to me that Sophocles recognizes that the truth, when it is fully revealed, is too terrible to be endured and that through his self-mutilation Oedipus is already in retreat from it.

The self-blinding of Oedipus

As the play approaches its climax, Jocasta, who has finally recognized the truth, rushes into the palace leaving Oedipus to interrogate the shepherd, who ultimately reveals the whole story. Now Oedipus, who has shown such ambivalence in his search for the truth, accepts it with great courage and without prevarication or excuse. He simply says, 'Alas! All out! All known! No more concealment! Oh light! May I never look on you again, revealed as I am, sinful in my begetting, sinful in marriage, sinful in shedding of blood.'

With these words he goes into the palace after Jocasta and, although he is faced with overwhelming guilt, at this point he fully acknowledges it and seems able to bear it. We are left to wait outside with the Chorus of Elders until, some time later, a messenger appears from within and we finally hear what has happened. It is immediately clear that a profound change has taken place, and what was an atmosphere of distress and pain gives way to one of horror. The messenger begins by saying,

Oh you most honourable lords of the city of Thebes, weep for the things you shall hear, the things you must see. . . . Not all the waters of Ister, the waters of Phasis, can wash this dwelling clean of the foulness within, clean of the deliberate acts that soon shall be

122

known, of all horrible acts most horrible, wilfully chosen. . . . First and in brief Her Majesty is dead.

These deliberate, wilfully chosen acts are the suicide of the Queen and the self-blinding of Oedipus, and they are described in terrible detail.

First we are told that Jocasta ran towards her marriage bed calling on Laius, and then that Oedipus roamed about the palace shouting for a sword. "'A sword, a sword!" he cried; "Where is that wife, no wife of mine – that soil where I was sown, and whence I reaped my harvest!'" The messenger continues,

> With wild hallooing cries he hurled himself upon the locked doors, bending by main force the bolts out of their sockets – and stumbled in. We saw a knotted pendulum, a noose, a strangled woman swinging before our eyes. The King saw too and with heart-rendering groans untied the rope, and laid her on the ground. But worse was yet to see. Her dress was pinned with golden brooches, which the King snatched out and thrust, from full arm's length, into his eyes – eyes that should see no longer his shame, his guilt, no longer see those they should never have seen, nor see, unseeing, those he had longed to see, henceforth seeing nothing but night. . . . To this wild tune he pierced his eyeballs time and time again till bloody tears ran down his beard – not drops but in full spate a whole cascade descending in drenching cataracts of scarlet rain. Thus two have sinned; and on two heads, not one – on man and wife – falls mingled punishment.

We are moved to horror and pity by these descriptions as we recognize that guilt has turned to hatred and hatred to tragic self-mutilation. Earlier, as the play moved towards its climax, we saw a gradual and hesitant journey towards the truth as Oedipus struggled to overcome his own and Jocasta's reluctance to accept it. Then he faces it fully for that brave but brief acknowledgement while Jocasta has gone into the palace, but at some point he can bear it no longer and his guilt turns to hatred.

It is clear that when Oedipus calls for a sword he intends to threaten and even kill Jocasta, and there is little doubt that he is already full of hatred towards her, probably because he realizes, on the evidence of the shepherd, that she was an accomplice to the attempt to kill him as a baby (Rudnytsky 1987). Perhaps his hatred of Jocasta starts with this recognition of her loyalty to Laius and her collusion in the wish to destroy him. However, her suicide is an even more catastrophic betrayal and adds the weight of Jocasta's death to the already heavy burden of his guilt. Both events lead to the realization that he has lost her as an ally who could help him bear his guilt and as an accomplice

123

who should share it with him. Now he has truly lost her, and I believe it is this loss which made the guilt unbearable and led Oedipus to turn his hatred first against Jocasta and next against himself.

Most significantly, he attacks his eyes, which are his link to the reality he cannot bear, and he tries to annihilate the source of his pain by destroying his capacity to experience and perceive. Later he explains that he would also have made himself deaf if he had been able to. 'Had I any way to dam that channel too, I would not rest till I had imprisoned up this body of shame in total blankness. For the mind to dwell beyond the reach of pain were peace indeed.'

When Oedipus emerges from the palace the Chorus are appalled at what he has done. They say, 'Ah! Horror beyond all bearing! Foulest disfigurement that ever I saw! O cruel, insensate agony! What demon of destiny with swift assault outstriding has ridden you down? . . . Those eyes – how could you do what you have done? What evil power had driven you to this end?' Their horror recognizes the enormity of the act of self-mutilation which makes it impossible to make reparation and to begin atonement, an act even worse than the original crimes of incest and parricide.

I believe these observations can help us to clarify the nature of Oedipal guilt and to think about what makes it bearable or unbearable (Steiner 1990a). It is normal for a child to have the phantasy that he can rid himself of his father in order to possess his mother, and the guilt for such phantasies only really becomes overwhelming when the full extent of the Oedipal crime is revealed. What horrifies the child is that, instead of being delighted that she now has her little son in place of her husband, his mother is shattered by the Oedipal murder, and the attack is revealed to be against both parents and against their relationship.

Indeed, although the actual crime may appear as parricide, it is often the child's mother who is hated more intensely because of the way she stimulates his desire and then betrays him by preferring his father. Other sources of hatred of the mother become revealed when her death becomes part of the Oedipal phantasy – in particular, envy of the breast as the primal good object.

We can also see how his mother's death seems to be unexpected and somehow doubly shocking for Oedipus. His father's murder and the marriage were, after all, part of the prophecy, but nowhere is Oedipus warned that his crime will devastate and destroy his mother too. No oracle proclaimed that he would kill his mother by driving her to suicide. He can claim that it was never his intention to devastate her, only to possess her, and until he sees her dead body, he could argue that he loved his mother and it was indeed this love which led to the Oedipal crimes. The horror and shock seem to take him completely by surprise and this kind of guilt seems unfair, and as it becomes unbearable it turns to hatred and despair.

Oedipus the King ends as Oedipus begs to be banished from Thebes in order that he will no longer pollute the city. Sophocles takes up the story again in *Oedipus at Colonus*, written perhaps twenty years later, and we find that not only has Oedipus survived but that he is once again going to triumph. This time he turns to omnipotence and is able to defeat his inner despair by becoming a holy man. It is a manic triumph which frightens us by its power and ruthlessness, and which impresses us through its grandeur. But in Vellacott's (1978) view, which I find most convincing, it is a retreat from truth, a retreat from contact with inner reality, and an abandonment of human values.

The story of *Oedipus at Colonus*

We meet Oedipus in this play as a blind old man wandering through the countryside, led by his faithful daughter Antigone. He has finally been banished from Thebes but only after a long delay and he is looking for somewhere to die. Both his daughters have given up their lives for him. Antigone guides and supports him in his journey, and Ismene stays at home looking after his interests there. By contrast, his two sons, Eteocles and Polynices, have refused to help their father, and are about to fight each other for power in Thebes. Eteocles remains with Creon in the city while Polynices retreats to Argos, where he assembles an army.

Arriving at the hamlet of Colonus within a mile of the city of Athens where King Theseus rules, Oedipus has stumbled upon the grove of the Eumenides, and the Elders of Colonus are horrified that he should enter such sacred ground. Oedipus, however, sees this as a sign from the god, since he has been promised by Apollo that he will find sanctuary and an end to his suffering in a holy place. The Elders are even more appalled when they discover who Oedipus is, and it is clear that his story is well known. They insist that he leave, and when Antigone pleads for him on compassionate grounds, they reply that they pity her but fear their own gods. Oedipus protests that he is innocent, and insists that he is a holy man who will bring great advantage to Athens. The Elders seem in awe of him and agree to his request that King Theseus be sent for.

In the meantime, Ismene arrives from Thebes carrying the news of the conflict between her brothers but also of a new decree from Delphi which states that whosoever offers a sanctuary for the body of Oedipus will be favoured by the gods and protected in battle. Oedipus is consequently now sought for by Polynices, but also by Creon who

125

wants him brought home and buried, close to the border of his city. His sin is not forgotten and he cannot actually enter Thebes, but will nevertheless protect it if buried nearby.

When Theseus arrives, Oedipus offers his body as a gift to Athens in exchange for a sanctuary for his grave within that very sacred grove at Colonus. Theseus, like the Elders, seems in awe of him and agrees. Creon appears, demanding the return of Oedipus, who responds with passionate hatred, with vehement protestations of innocence, and with righteous anger. Creon tries to take him by force and has already abducted his daughters but the Elders intervene and Theseus returns to save Oedipus and subsequently to free Ismene and Antigone. Next Polynices comes to plead with his father and is rejected and cursed with a terrible coldness as Oedipus refuses to soften despite the protestations of Theseus and Antigone.

Finally, Oedipus prepares himself for death and glory because of his special religious significance. Only Theseus will know the precise place of his burial, and this secret will be handed down to the subsequent rulers of Athens who will in this way ensure its invulnerability.

If we compare the character of Oedipus as we see it in this play with that portrayed in *Oedipus the King* we cannot but be impressed with the change in him. We no longer see a man who could acknowledge his guilt and who was subsequently shattered by the discovery of the true nature of the Oedipal crime, but instead we meet a haughty, arrogant man who makes repeated and devious self-excuses, who adopts a superior grandeur and relates to others including his sons with coldness and cruelty, and who in taking on divine characteristics sheds the very humanity he fought so hard to achieve (Vellacott 1978).

This is clear, first of all, in the protestations of innocence which Oedipus repeats again and again with vehemence and self-righteousness. For example, while addressing the Elders of Colonus he says:

'My strength has been in suffering, not doing — as you should hear, could I but tell it; could tell all that my father and my mother did — whence comes, I know your fear. Was I the sinner? Repaying wrong for wrong — that was no sin, even were it wittingly done, as it was not. I did not know the way I went. They knew; they who devised this trap for me, they knew!'

When the Chorus points out later that he had after all killed his father, Oedipus replies that he had done so with justice: 'Yes with justice. You shall hear. He whom I killed had sought to kill me first. The law acquits me, innocent, as ignorant of what I did.'

In his argument with Creon he defends himself as follows:

'My life was innocent, search as you will of any guilty secret for which this error could have been the punishment, this sin that damned myself and all my blood. Or tell me: if my father was foredoomed by the voice of heaven to die by his own son's hand, how can you justly cast it against me, who was still unborn when that decree was spoken? Nay unbegotten, unconceived. And if being born, as I was for this calamity, I chanced to meet my father and to kill him, not knowing who he was or what I did – how can you hold the unwitting crime against me?'

He proceeds:

'Yet this I must say again! I am not condemned, and shall not be, either for my marrying or for my father's murder, which your spite persists in casting in my teeth. Answer me this one thing: if here and now someone came up and threatened to take your life, your innocent life, would you then pause to ask if he were your father – or deal with him out of hand? I am sure as you love life you'd pay the assailant in his own coin, not look for legal warrant. Such by the god's contrivance was my case. My father himself, if he could live again, would not deny it.'

Vellacott points out that these arguments have to be taken in their context since, if you have just been told by an oracle that you are destined to kill your father, then you might indeed hesitate if a man of your father's age threatened you. Moreover, the protestations are inconsistent. If you do not know who it is you are killing it cannot also be a defence that you are justified because your father tried to kill you when you were a baby. Oedipus seems to be saying, 'I am not to blame because he struck me first, I am not to blame because I did not know who it was I killed or whom I married, and finally I am justified because they tried to have me killed as a baby!'

The previous admission of responsibility and guilt is replaced by a haughty coldness and by a grandeur which derives from his assumption that he is pure and holy. The conviction that he is right which gives such confidence to his anger comes out in his quarrel with Creon, but most of all in the rejection of his son. He curses Polynices, not for making war on his own city, Thebes, nor because he is threatening to destroy his own brother, but because he did not help Oedipus when he was banished. With implacable hatred he proclaims,

'And take this malediction in your ears; may you never defeat your motherland; may you never return alive to Argos; may you, in dying, kill your banisher, and, killing, die by him who shares your blood. This is my prayer.'

Thus both sons are cursed in a mood reminiscent of the hatred Laius must have felt, a generation earlier, for the infant Oedipus.

Although we are chilled at the righteous anger and coldness of Oedipus, we recognize the appalling nature of the guilt he has to carry, and as we become aware that it is impossible to stay in touch with such unbearable feelings, we feel pity and compassion for Oedipus. Human feelings such as these are aroused in the audience listening to the play, and they contrast sharply with the hostility, hatred, and stubbornness of Oedipus. These human feelings are represented above all in the character of Antigone, who tries to get him to soften his hatred for his son Polynices.

> 'You are his father; and it cannot be right, even if he has done you the cruellest, wickedest wrong, for you to do him wrong again. Let him come. Many a father has wayward sons to vex him, but soothing friends can charm them out of anger. Forget the present, and remember the old hard things that happened to you on account of your father and mother. Will they not remind you what evil consequences come out of angry impulse? I think they must with the lesson of your sightless eyes.'

Vellacott argues that Sophocles uses Antigone to discuss the nature and origin of morality itself. Where can it begin, if not in recognizing as absolute, the authority of reverence for kindred blood? If that authority can be set aside because of special circumstances, what other moral authority has any hope of becoming established (Vellacott 1978)? Here the principle of loyalty to the family is shown in direct conflict with the law of retaliation. The play balances the authority of the holy as represented by Oedipus with the authority of the good in Antigone.

In contrast to the humanity of Antigone, we see how Oedipus idealizes a moral severity based on the law of the talion, an eye for an eye and a tooth for a tooth. As he raises himself to the stature of a god it becomes less and less appropriate for him to feel guilt. Gods are familiar with wrath, but they can admit no wrong and guilt is foreign to them.

Oedipus had to face death, and in the process he is brought into contact with the deepest of anxieties as he enters the unknown and says goodbye to those who have sustained him in life, in particular his family. To say goodbye is to face loss, and in this way facing one's own death also involves mourning. Vellacott argues that it is man's mortality, the knowledge that he must die, which creates in him the moral dimension which gods lack. I believe it is this moral dimension which results from the act of mourning as we face the reality of death. It is the pain and guilt which has to be faced in these confrontations with reality which are so difficult to bear and which can lead to a *retreat from truth to omnipotence*.

128

To conclude, I want to compare briefly the way Oedipus dealt with reality in the period up to his blinding, when I suggest the chief mechanism was that of *turning a blind eye*, with that in the period described in *Colonus* which followed his banishment, when it seemed that he turned to omnipotence and self-righteousness.

Two methods of evading reality

Mechanisms such as *turning a blind eye* which keep facts conveniently out of sight and allow someone to know and not to know simultaneously can be highly pathological and lead to distortions and misrepresentations of the truth, but it is important to recognize that they still reflect a respect and a fear of the truth and it is this fear which leads to the collusion and the cover-up. This mechanism is related to those used for dealing with the truth in perversions and can be thought of as a perversion of the truth leading to distortions and misrepresentations of it. Oedipus adopts a state of mind which can be thought of as a psychic retreat from reality and a defence against anxiety and guilt. The retreat was based on a pathological organization which involved objects in a collusion to deny reality each with their own separate motives. It seemed to have served him well until the plague, possibly representing the corruption which was covered up, led him to begin his struggle to face the truth. Perhaps like a mid-life crisis (Jaques 1965), reality caught up with him as he had to face problems which were incompletely dealt with earlier.

In *Oedipus at Colonus*, Oedipus, now actually blind, can no longer *turn a blind eye*, and instead turns to authority, in fact divine authority, and in this way gains the persuasive power and moral conviction which enable him to show a contempt for the truth. He does not deny the facts themselves, it is too late to pretend that he did not kill his father and marry his mother, but he denies responsibility and guilt, and claims that these acts were wrongs inflicted *on* him rather than by him. The gods who singled him out to perpetrate the most awful acts now promise to make him a hero and elevate him to the status of near god (Winnington-Ingram 1980). He no longer shows a respect for reality, and the retreat to omnipotence makes it inappropriate to feel shame or to try to conceal his crimes.

This kind of relationship to reality is based on a *retreat from truth to omnipotence* and is clearly very different from that of *turning a blind eye*. The retreat is one in which reality is dismissed and the organization on which it is based is peopled with omnipotent figures who claim respect from their divinity and power. The truth does not have to be argued

129

or justified and shame and guilt are inappropriate. It is indeed the lack of shame which makes these alliances with omnipotent figures so dangerous since normal restraints on destructiveness and cruelty are rendered inoperative.

This kind of alliance arises when something has gone radically wrong in the relationship with primary objects in the nuclear family. It is these figures – chiefly the parents, of course – which make up the normal superego, and because it results from the internalization of human figures, the normal superego is a human one with ordinary human hopes and fears. If these objects are destroyed, or if the parental imagos are too distorted by the projection of primitive sadism, a more primitive, powerful, and cruel superego will result (Klein 1932). If the guilt becomes unbearable, self-mutilating attacks on the perceiving ego may be resorted to and the resulting damage leaves a disability which can only be patched over by means of omnipotence since ordinary human figures are too weak to be of help.

The individual is then possessed by more monstrous forces, and since these contain projected parts of the self a complex structure results. Here too we have a pathological organization of the personality, but one organized at a more primitive level. Whereas all pathological organizations are basically narcissistic in structure, they differ markedly in form. When they take on a paranoid grandiosity, as in *Oedipus at Colonus*, they seem to protect the individual from paranoid-schizoid disintegration and fragmentation. Sometimes the psychotic character of the retreat, and of the organization underlying it, is obvious, but at times of crisis its psychotic nature may be more difficult to recognize. At these times omnipotence is so much sought after by all of us that we are ready to accept as a hero what in normal circumstances we would recognize as a madman.

Vellacott suggests that Sophocles has, throughout the play, separated the *sacred* from the *good*. At times of crisis the good is treated as a weakness which we cannot afford because survival demands a reliance on powerful gods whose sanctity must not be questioned. We are fortunate then if the *good* can be located in a group or an individual where it might survive until it can again be recognized. Near the end of *Colonus*, the Chorus liken Oedipus to 'A rock in a wild north sea at winter's height, fronting the rude assault of all the billows of adversity that break upon his head from every side unceasing'. It is clear that for him *strength* is a priority, and what remains of hope lies in Antigone who pleads to Theseus, 'Then pray you see us safe returned to age-old Thebes. There it may be we can yet stem the tide of blood that dooms our brothers.'

11

Problems of psychoanalytic technique: patient-centred and analyst-centred interpretations

Patients who withdraw excessively to psychic retreats present major problems of technique. The frustration of having a stuck patient, who is at the same time out of reach, challenges the analyst, who has to avoid being driven either to give up in despair or to over-react and try to overcome opposition and resistance in too forceful a way. The situation is one where the patient and analyst can easily be at cross purposes. The patient is interested in regaining or retaining his equilibrium, which is achieved by a withdrawal to a psychic retreat, while the analyst is concerned to help the patient emerge, to help him gain insight into the way his mind works, and to allow development to proceed.

Joseph (1983) has pointed out that the patient, in this state of mind, is not interested in understanding, and uses the analysis for a variety of purposes other than that of gaining insight into his problems. In these circumstances his main concern is to obtain relief and security by establishing a mental equilibrium and in consequence he is unable to direct his interest towards understanding. The priority for the patient is to get rid of unwanted mental contents, which he projects into the analyst, and in these states he is able to take very little back into his mind. He does not have the time or the space to think, and he is afraid to examine his own mental processes. Words are used, not primarily to convey information, but as actions having an effect on the analyst, and the analyst's words are likewise felt as actions indicating something about the analyst's state of mind rather than offering insight to the patient. If the analyst believes his task is to help the patient gain understanding and if the patient is unwilling or unable to tolerate such understanding, then an impasse is likely. Such situations are not uncommon and present distressing problems for patient and analyst alike.

Throughout this book I have discussed different ways in which contact with the analyst, and with reality, can be evaded, distorted, and misrepresented, and I have described how various mechanisms are brought into play when reality is unbearable. When these mechanisms are welded into a pathological organization of the personality which provides a retreat from reality, the analyst may be tolerated only if he submits to the rules imposed by the organization. Pressure is put on him to agree to the limits which the patient sets on what is tolerable, and this may mean that certain types of interpretation are either not permitted or not listened to. If the analyst becomes too insistent that his task is to help the patient gain insight and develop, an even more obstinate withdrawal to the retreat may result and an impasse can materialize which is extremely difficult to negotiate. If, on the other hand, the analyst takes too passive a stance, the patient may feel he has given up, and may see the analyst as defeated or dishonestly caught up in a collusion with a perverse organization.

The formidable technical problems which arise from this situation are, in part, therefore, due to the uncomfortable counter-transference feelings which are evoked in the analyst. The patient is usually acutely aware of the discomfort in the analyst but is unable to recognize his role in the creation of the situation and is unaware or unconcerned with his own internal problems. The analyst's interpretations are felt as intrusions threatening his place in the retreat, and he fears that if he emerges from its protection he faces either persecutory disintegration or unbearable depressive pain.

In this chapter I want to make a distinction between *understanding* and *being understood*, and point out that the patient who is not interested in acquiring understanding – that is, understanding about himself – may yet have a pressing need to be understood by the analyst. Sometimes this is consciously experienced as a wish to be understood, and sometimes it is unconsciously communicated. A few patients appear to hate the whole idea of being understood and try to disavow it and get rid of all meaningful contact. Even this kind of patient, however, needs the analyst to register what is happening and to have his situation and his predicament recognized.

The transference is often loaded with anxiety which the patient is unable to contend with but which has to be contained in the analytic situation, and such containment depends on the analyst's capacity to recognize and cope with what the patient has projected and with his own counter-transference reactions to it. Experience suggests that such containment is weakened if the analyst perseveres in interpreting or explaining to the patient what he is thinking, feeling, or doing. The patient experiences such interpretations as a lack of containment and feels that the analyst is pushing the projected elements back into him. He has projected these precisely because he could not cope with them and his immediate need is for them to continue to reside in the analyst and to be understood in their projected state.

Some analysts, in these circumstances, tend to phrase their interpretations in a form which recognizes that the patient is more interested in what is going on in the *analyst's* mind than in his own. At these times the patient's most immediate concern is his experience of the analyst, and this can be addressed by saying something like, 'You experience me as . . .', or 'You are afraid that I . . .', or 'You were relieved when I . . .', or 'You became anxious a moment ago when I . . .'. I think of such interpretations as *analyst-centred* and differentiate them from *patient-centred* interpretations, which are of the classical kind in which something the patient is doing, thinking, or wishing is interpreted, often together with the motive and the anxiety associated with it. In general, patient–centred interpretations are more concerned with conveying understanding, whereas analyst–centred interpretations are more likely to give the patient a sense of being understood.

Of course, the distinction between the two types of transference interpretation is schematic, and in a deeper sense all interpretations are centred on the patient and reflect the analyst's attempt to understand the patient's experience. The problem is to recognize where the patient's anxieties and preoccupations are focused. In practice, most interpretations take into account both what the patient feels and what he thinks the analyst feels and include a reference to both patient and analyst. When we say, 'You experience me as . . .' or 'You are afraid that I . . .', a *patient-centred* element is present because we are talking about the patient's 'experience' and 'fear'. Moreover, it is clear that the distinction depends more on the analyst's attitude and state of mind than on the wording he uses. If the analyst says, 'You see me as . . .' and implies that the patient's view is one which is in error, or hurtful, or in some other way undesirable, then the emphasis is on what is going on in the patient and the interpretation is primarily patient-centred. To be analyst-centred, in the sense which I intend to use it, the analyst has to have an open mind and be willing to consider the patient's view and try to understand what the patient means in a spirit of enquiry. Although these considerations complicate the distinction between the two types of interpretation and suggest gradations between them I will consider them to be distinct for the sake of clarity. Both types of interpretations are necessary for the patient's total situation to be understood and both types have dangers attached to them if they are used excessively and without due attention to the feedback the patient gives about his reaction to them.

133

Sometimes the *patient-centred* element is elaborated further, and we may say something like 'You are *trying* to get me to feel . . . such and such', or, 'Your attack on me just now gave rise to such and such a result'. The interpretation then involves a *link* between what the patient does, thinks, or wishes, and the state of the analyst. Sometimes these links take the form of a *because* clause which is added to an *analyst-centred* interpretation. We may say, 'You are afraid that I am upset *because* of the fact that you did such and such.' Such links are the essence of deep analytic work but are particularly difficult for the patient who is caught up in a pathological organization of the personality. They imply that he is not only capable of taking an interest in his own actions but able to accept responsibility for them as well, and this implies a degree of independence which challenges the dominance of the organization. It is especially in these patients and in the early stages of an analysis that it is necessary to recognize the problems which ensue from both types of interpretation and from the links which arise between them.

Clinical material

I believe that the distinction between these two types of transference interpretation can help the analyst to examine the technical problems he has been struggling with and may allow him to shift from one type of interpretation to the other when it appears to be appropriate. In order to examine these issues I will first briefly look again at the material from a psychotic patient (Mr C) which I have discussed in greater detail in Chapter 6.

This patient was very paranoid and concrete in his thinking, and spoke with triumph about his ability to hurt the analyst which he connected with the way he hurt his mother when she had a breast infection when he was a baby. He then announced his intention to change his job, which meant ending his analysis, which made the analyst feel sad at the idea of losing his patient. This led the analyst to make a patient–centred interpretation, saying that the patient wanted to get rid of his own sadness and wanted *him*, the analyst, to feel the pain of separation and loss. The patient said, 'Yes, I can do to you what you do to me. You are in my hands. There is an equalization.' A moment later he started to complain that he was being poisoned, and after discussing government policies of nuclear deterrence he complained of gastric troubles and diarrhoea and explained that he had to shit out every word the analyst gave him in order not to be contaminated by infected milk.

It seems to me that the patient found the patient–centred interpretation to be threatening because it exposed him to experiences such as grief, anxiety, and guilt, which were associated with the loss of his analyst. He felt that the interpretation had forced him to take these feelings back into himself and he experienced them concretely as poison and tried to evacuate them in his faeces. The patient indicated the catastrophic nature of his anxiety by talking about nuclear disaster. He needed the analyst to recognize that he could maintain a relationship with him only if the analyst agreed to hold the experiences associated with loss in his own mind and to refrain from trying to return these prematurely to the patient. After a transient contact with the experience of loss the psychotic process re-asserted itself in the patient's assertion that he would shit out every word the analyst said.

This is a situation where the interpretation may be unbearable even when it is correct. The psychotic process has made experience so concrete that insight is poison and has to be evacuated in faeces. When the analyst suggested that the patient wanted to get rid of his sadness and wanted the analyst to feel the pain of separation and loss, he was making a link between the patient's wishes and the analyst's state of mind. The patient felt that the analyst disapproved of these wishes and was himself pushing the distressed feelings back into the patient, and this led him to withdraw once more to the protection of the psychotic organization which asserted that disturbing insight was poison.

A different situation is seen when the patient is not psychotic and has a greater capacity to tolerate understanding and insight. This was the case in the material I will next discuss taken from the analysis of a 40-year-old academic woman (Mrs G) some two years after her analysis began. As a child she habitually withdrew to a phantasy world in which she joined figures from books or television to escape from the distress and anxiety going on in the family around her. The history contained many reports of extremely disturbed, wild, and even violent behaviour, and she often found herself in situations where she seemed to invite exploitation, mistreatment, and even danger. This was particularly true in her adolescence and was now being repeated by her 14-year-old daughter who created enormous problems for her.

After missing a Monday session she began on Tuesday by saying, 'I wondered if you would get the message. I spoke to a girl who said that she would put it in your drawer. I know what happens to messages like that. On Sunday I had wondered about ringing you at home.

'On the train I imagined meeting someone I know who would ask, "How are you?" I would reply, "Fine, only my department is collapsing, my daughter has run off and I don't know where she is, my husband is fed up and helpless and otherwise I am fine."'

She continued by explaining that she had missed Monday because of an important meeting with the university bursar to discuss finance which she decided she had to attend. She knew about this on the weekend and had wondered if she would phone to see if I could offer a different time. Instead she phoned my secretary early on Monday morning and, suspecting that the message would not reach me, had phoned again during her session time to explain that she was not coming. In fact it turned out that just before going into the meeting she was told it would be better if she did not attend and she said that they implied that she would be a liability. She added that there was something theatrical about the way her colleagues were behaving and that, as a result, the negotiation with the bursar was not straight-forward.

It is clear that we already have a complex communication and enactment between patient and analyst. There is a patient who wants to get a message through to her analyst and various obstacles come in the way. There is a woman who tells a friend that everything is fine but makes sure that she knows there are disasters all round, and there is a professor who tries to attend an important meeting but is told she is not wanted because she is a liability. These stories all have powerful transference implications which I believe centre on the patient's need to get through to the analyst that there is something very seriously wrong which needs attention. This need to get a message through is central to the interactions in the session but it is complicated by other motives. For example, it was possible to recognize a perverse side of her, which hated being understood, and which hindered or sabotaged communication, making everything far from straightforward. The imagined comment to the friend on the tube is not simply a message indicating how she feels, but is likely to make the person hearing it very uneasy, guilty, and confused.

In this situation I believe it is possible to concentrate our attention on either the patient's or the analyst's state of mind, mental mechanisms, and behaviour. Ultimately, the aim of an analysis is to help the patient gain an understanding of herself, and even in this material interpretations could have been used to explore the way she reacted and behaved. However, in this instance, I believe the patient was primarily concerned with the way her objects behaved. She felt that I did not make it easy for her to make contact with me on the weekend, and she had to overcome a feeling that she was a liability and unwanted if she intruded. Consciously she felt that she did her best and tried to get through to my secretary but she knew what happened to messages which are supposed to be left. When she imagined saying everything was fine she was partly being ironic, and partly trying to make me uncomfortable. Moreover, she left open the possibility that she was being theatrical, so that it was not clear what her inner reality was. I thought there were elements of despair and helplessness in the way she felt obliged to say she was fine and to go on coping somehow. The statement, although clearly a negation of feeling fine, left it open to the analyst to choose to ignore the irony and against all the evidence to hear her to mean that she *was* actually fine. She herself was sometimes convinced that this was the case and that it was other people who were making an unnecessary fuss. These thoughts led me to feel that despite the fact that she was not always able to carry out a straightforward negotiation she needed me to recognize her desperation and she feared that I would prefer to agree that everything was fine even though I knew very well that the contrary was true.

It would have been quite possible to use *patient-centred* interpretations and, for example, discuss the way she used irony, provocation, and passivity to create a situation where she was misunderstood, but I thought she would experience this as an attempt to make her responsible for her failure to get through to me, and that it would indicate my reluctance to accept responsibility for my contribution to the obstacles which stood in her way. In fact, it was probably true that her passivity and inability to fight for her needs helped to achieve the projection into me of guilt, pain, and responsibility. If so she would, in principle, benefit from an understanding of these mechanisms, which no doubt contributed to her difficulties, but I feared that she was in no state to be interested in understanding issues such as this. What she wanted was that I recognize that something was terribly wrong with her and that I accept the feelings this aroused in me and refrain from projecting them back into her. She was afraid that I was not going to be able to cope with these feelings because they would disturb *my* mental equilibrium.

I interpreted that she feared I was not able to create a setting where messages would get through to me, and I drew her attention to the atmosphere of the current session where she seemed relatively composed. I said that she hoped that I would see that beneath this composure things were very far from fine. However, I found myself saying that she also hinted that something theatrical was going on and I wondered if this was expressed in the way she tried to make contact. I suggested that this left her unsure if I could see through the theatricality to what she really felt.

After I had spoken I realized that this additional comment had a somewhat critical tone to it which I suspected arose from my difficulty in containing feelings, including those of anxiety, about her and possibly my annoyance that she made me feel responsible, guilty, and helpless. It is an example of a 'double-barrelled' interpretation in which the analyst is not content to make a single point but adds a second which is nearly always unnecessary and often unhelpful. In this instance I knew from past experience that a comment with a critical tinge could lead to the enactment of a sado-masochistic relationship in which she would feel the victim of an unfair attack and withdraw in silence.

She was silent for a while and then spoke of the fraught relationship she was having with her daughter. She described the way she wound everyone up and how she had screamed that she could not bear to live with them and had stormed out. At first she said it was for good, but later she phoned and said she would be back for school on Monday. In fact, she failed to turn up, and Mrs G had to ring the school and explain because they were also at the end of their tether with her and had threatened expulsion. She told them she knew it was terrible, but what could she do?

I considered this to be a comment on the interaction which had just taken place and a reaction to the interpretation I had made. At one level I thought she felt I had been critical, and like her daughter she had the impulse to withdraw in anger. It was difficult to know how to respond, but I thought it was probably better to refrain from emphasizing this side of the relationship. I did not think she would be able to take responsibility for her contribution to the difficulties in communication between us, and that interpreting them would probably feed a view of herself as an abused victim. I thought she disowned these feelings in the session and identified with me as a parent who could not cope.

It was thoughts like these which made me interpret that she needed me to accept the sense of helplessness when my patient disappears which may be something like her feeling when her daughter disappears. She needed me to cope with the anxiety associated with her not coming to her session and not being able to get in touch with me. She felt I blamed her for this just as she now feared I was too critical and defensive to understand her anger and disappointment with me and to recognize that she also wanted to make contact, she had not in fact withdrawn and did try to reach me and get through to me.

After a silence, she continued with more material about her daughter and the dangerous company of older criminal youths she was associating with. She described how she had tried to trace her by phoning her friends and their parents, and that when she had discovered this she was furious, abusing Mrs G and accusing her of spying on her and controlling her. She had also tried to get her ex-husband, her adoptive father, to go and bring her home but he said he was busy and had no car. He thought the girl should be allowed to find her own way back in her own time.

This made a direct connection with my own experience of her behaviour in the session. I thought that she was identified with her role as a helpless mother but that the angry, disturbed patient who was furious with me, who could not bear to be with me, and who had such difficulties in getting through to me was not directly available. This was a familiar problem and left me uncertain if I should try to pursue her or wait for her to return.

I interpreted that she saw me as helpless when she withdrew and was afraid that I would leave it to her to find her way back to the session. This made her fear that I did not take the danger she was in seriously. I did, however, add a patient–centred element when I said that, if I did try to reach her when she felt disturbed, violent, and out of control, she made it clear that, like her daughter, she would be angry and feel intruded on and controlled.

The remainder of the session continued in similar vein. She described how her colleagues had to put on an act with the bursar to persuade him that the department was in a terrible financial state but that with applicants and colleagues from other universities the problem was exactly the opposite since *they* had to be convinced that the department was viable. There were references to the real possibility of being closed down and to the necessity of making staff redundant in order to avoid this. I had a strong impression of her insecurity, and because of numerous recent hints that she might not be able to continue her analysis, of my own possible redundancy. These themes linked with her need to fit in with the way her colleagues worked even when she disapproved of their methods. It corresponded to an internal situation where she felt trapped in an organization she hated but at the same time felt she needed and could not extricate herself from.

This session was fairly typical in terms of the anxiety she generated, and also showed both the problems she had in staying in touch with it and the problems she generated in me. If I tried to make contact with a very disturbed patient who found it difficult to come to the session, she felt that I pursued her and she made it clear that she would not tolerate that. If, on the other hand, I was too passive, if I seemed to throw up my hands as she did and claim that there was nothing more I could do, she was afraid that I would give up and see the analysis as bankrupt and hopeless. If I made *patient-centred* interpretations, she felt intruded upon and experienced it as my failure to cope with the anxiety which led to my blaming her and pushing the anxiety back into her. I thought she tolerated *analyst-centred* interpretations better, but she sometimes saw them as a confession that I was not coping and as an admission that I was afraid to tackle her difficulties and face the consequences.

Discussion

Technical problems such as those I encountered in this material can be thought of as expressions of the patient's resistance, on the one hand, and of the analyst's counter-transference difficulties, on the other. Our understanding of both of these has been enhanced as we learn more about the mechanism of projective identification (Klein 1946; Rosenfeld 1971b), and about *containment* (Bion 1959, 1962a, 1963) and *counter-transference* (Heimann 1950, 1960; Money-Kyrle 1956; Racker 1957; Sandler 1976), which are closely related to it.

Both Sandler (1976) and Joseph (1981) have recognized the way in which patients nudge and prod the analyst in order to create a particular situation in the transference. Sandler describes how an internal relationship between the self and an object becomes *actualized* in the relationship with the analyst, who is led to enact an *infantile role-relationship*. As a counterpart to Freud's *free-floating attention*, he points out that the analyst has to have a *free-floating responsiveness* and that the analyst's reactions as well as his thoughts and feelings contribute to his counter-transference. Joseph shows how it is through such *enactments* that the analyst is drawn into playing a role in the patient's phantasy and as a result is used as part of his defensive system. The patient may of course interpret such actualizations and infantile role-relationships in a delusional way and come to believe that they were achieved not by natural means but by omnipotent phantasy.

We have come to use counter-transference to refer to the totality of the analyst's reactions in his relationship with the patient. The recognition of the importance of projective identification in creating these reactions led naturally to the idea that counter-transference is an important source of information about the state of mind of the patient. The analyst can try to observe his own reactions to the patient and to the totality of the situation in the session and to use them to understand what the patient is projecting into him.

But counter-transference also has its problems when we come to try to use it in practice, perhaps most of all because the analyst's introspection is complicated by his own defensive needs so that many important counter-transference reactions remain unconscious. Self-deception and unconscious collusion with the patient to evade reality makes counter-transference unreliable without additional corroboration. Here a third point of view can help the analyst to recognize his blind spots and fortify his judgements (Segal 1991; Britton 1989). The analyst may use colleagues and supervisors whom he can consult between sessions and whose presence he can to some degree internalize. Most of all he can use the help which his patient gives, sometimes through a direct criticism of his work, but more often through his reactions to the interpretations he has given.

Because of the propensity to be nudged into enactments with the patient it is often impossible to understand exactly what has been happening at the moment when it is taking place. Sandler (1976) suggests that the analyst may catch a counter-transference reaction within himself, particularly if it is in the direction of being inappropriate, but he recognizes that such self-awareness may only occur after the responses have been carried over into action. In either case it is clear that immediate counter-transference reactions have to be reviewed a few minutes later when the patient's reaction is available, and this may have to be repeated as further understanding develops later in the session or in subsequent sessions. Using all the means available to him, including his self-observation, the observation of his actions, the responses of the patient and the overall atmosphere of the session, the analyst can arrive at some kind of understanding of his patient and of his interaction with him. If he can stand the pressure he is put under, he can use this understanding to formulate an interpretation which allows the patient to feel understood and contained. When this is convincing, the patient feels that the analyst can contain those elements he has projected into him and as a result the projected elements become more bearable. The patient feels relief and is able to use the analyst's capacity to think, feel, and experience, in order to help him cope.

If the analyst is *unable* to contain the projections and closes himself off or counter-projects, the patient feels attacked and misunderstood and is likely to become increasingly disturbed and to intensify the splitting and the projective mechanisms he has been using. On the other hand, successful containment leads to integration, and the experience of being understood may then provide a context where further development can take place.

Such further development is necessary for lasting psychic change to occur, and, in my view, it does not automatically follow containment but depends on the acquisition of insight and understanding by the patient. Successful containment, which is associated with being understood rather than with acquiring understanding, is a necessary but not a sufficient condition for these developments. Containment requires that the projected elements have been able to enter the analyst's mind, where they can be registered and given meaning which is convincing. It does not require that the patient himself is available or interested in achieving understanding. If the patient is to develop further, he must make a fundamental shift, and develop an interest in understanding, no matter how small or fleeting. This kind of shift, which reflects the beginning of a capacity to tolerate insight and mental pain, is associated with a move from the paranoid–schizoid to the depressive position. I will try and illustrate how such a development depends on the experience of separateness and loss in a further fragment of clinical material.

A further clinical fragment

A few months following the sessions described above, the patient was told that I was taking an extra week's break in mid-term. She usually dealt with such disruptions in routine by missing a few sessions, partly in revenge but mostly, I thought, to serve as a means of projecting the experience of being left, into me. This time she began a session by describing how she had walked to work as usual with her husband and passed a neighbour's house where she saw that a light was on in an attic room. She knew that this room had been recently converted to house the family's new baby and as they passed she imagined one of the parents attending to the baby. This made her wonder if it really was too late for her to have a baby with her present husband, and she shuddered as she thought of all the gynaecological problems which would have to be overcome and which had led to so many complications and to endless painful investigations in her first pregnancy. They turned a corner and she passed the street where her colleague and chief rival lived. She had a very difficult relationship with this woman whom she admired but also felt controlled by, and she described how, normally, when she passed she would look right into the house and would often see her colleague moving around choosing what she was going to wear that day. On this occasion, however, she could not see into the house clearly because tears were in her eyes.

I interpreted that while she reacted to my week off in various ways she seemed today to associate this with the idea that I had other things to attend to, like a baby, and that this put her in touch with her grief and made her feel more separate and tearful. Her mood was quiet and thoughtful and we could use the session to explore how previously she dealt with separations by entering my mind just as she used to enter her colleague's house, her family and her department.

Periods of contact like this were not frequent and were not sustained, but they did give rise to moments when she seemed genuinely interested in the way her mind worked and was consequently able to accept *patient-centred* interpretations. On this occasion the shift was associated with the patient's sadness when she feared that she no longer had the mental and physical capacity to have a baby of her own. She felt more separate from me, and her tears enabled her to accept a momentary contact with a psychic reality. This small and transient shift to the depressive position allowed her to become interested in her own mind and her own mental processes.

Further discussion

In psychotic and borderline patients, as well as others functioning at a paranoid–schizoid level, containment brings relief but does not necessarily lead to growth and development. One of the reasons for this is that the relief depends on the continuing presence of the containing object since, at this level of organization, true separateness from the object cannot be tolerated and, as a result, the capacity to contain cannot yet be internalized. The object has been incorporated into the organization so that the threat of its loss leads to panic and to the deployment of omnipotent phantasy to create the illusion that the object is possessed and controlled. The patient internalizes an object containing the projected elements and does not truly face the experience of separateness. Sometimes such omnipotent phantasies are delusional and survive all evidence to the contrary, but in most cases contrary evidence is more subtly evaded and experiences such as the regular timing of sessions fuel the patient's illusion that his analyst is not free to act independently and unexpectedly.

This was illustrated by the way my patient ordinarily dealt with separations by projective identification, which she experienced as entering my mind and body where she was able to control me but where she also saw herself as inside me and hence as my responsibility. In the first section of the clinical material, I tried to show how difficult she was to contain when this happened. Her wild, dangerous, and aggressive behaviour was subtly hidden behind her composure but was apparent when I had such trouble finding and reaching her. My worries about her were paralleled in the terrible worries she had about her daughter. When I was able to contain her anxiety about my ability to cope with such responsibility she seemed relieved. But this relief needed the analyst's presence to act as a container and could survive beyond the end of the session only through a denial of separateness. Such denial was associated with a possessive hold of her objects which remained under her omnipotent control.

Inevitably, occasions arise when the analyst temporarily steps outside the patient's omnipotent control and a degree of separateness is achieved. This seemed to take place in the session I reported soon after I announced an unexpected break in the analysis, and was connected with a recognition that it was her neighbour and not herself who had the baby she so much wanted. My freedom to act was associated with a lessening of omnipotent control and led to an experience of loss which enabled her to feel more separate and in the process to express some of her sadness and grief which, I think, made up part of the work of mourning her lost objects and lost opportunities. I have argued elsewhere (Chapters 4 and 5, in particular) that it is through the work of mourning that the patient is able to regain those parts of herself which she previously got rid of through projective identification, and that with further work these projected fragments can be reintegrated in the ego (Steiner 1990a).

It is at these times that the patient could take a true interest into her own mind and begin to differentiate what belonged to the analyst and what belonged to her. Such moves towards the depressive position are clearly more frequent in less disturbed patients and at later stages of an analysis, but they may occur at any time even if only for brief and isolated moments. They require a prior capacity on the part of the analyst to contain and integrate the projected elements, but I believe that they also demand that the analyst have the courage to take risks and, when appropriate, give a *patient-centred* interpretation even if this may lead to a persecuted patient.

Shifting between the two types of interpretation

In the clinical material I presented I tried to be sensitive to the need to shift between the two types of interpretation, and I encountered problems with both. When I focused on the patient's behaviour and, for example, interpreted her theatricality or her withdrawal into silence, she felt intruded upon and blamed for the failure to make contact with me. It was when *patient-centred* interpretations implied that she was responsible for what happened between us that she became most persecuted and tended to withdraw. It was particularly over the question of responsibility that she felt I sometimes adopted a righteous tone which made her feel that I was refusing to examine my own contribution to the problem and unwilling to accept responsibility myself. In the counter-transference this issue created serious problems for me, since, when the patient projected feelings with such intensity, I often felt that I was being made responsible for the patient's problems as well as my own.

It is in such situations that I believe it may be better to be sparing with the *patient-centred* elements in the interpretation, to concentrate on the patient's view of the analyst, and to avoid making premature links between the two. Of course this is not a formula which can be used to solve technical problems, and, as we have seen, *analyst-centred* interpretations have their own difficulties. They too can fail to offer containment, sometimes because they are simply wrong and out of touch and sometimes because the patient feels the analyst is interpreting to cover up his situation rather than to confront it. Too many *analyst-centred* interpretations make the patient feel that the analyst is preoccupied with himself and unable to observe and respond to the patient and his problems. Moreover, sometimes this view of the analyst is justified. The patient is always listening for information about the analyst's state of mind, and whatever form of interpretation he uses, verbal and non-verbal clues give the patient information about him. The patient can use these to see if what the analyst says matches how he expresses himself, and this is important in his view of the analyst's character and trustworthiness.

Sometimes interpreting the patient's view of the analyst helps the patient recognize that he has projected an archaic internal figure into him and is expecting the analyst to behave, say, as his mother would have behaved. The interpretation may clarify this and enable the patient to see the analyst subsequently in a different light. Sometimes, however, the interpretation simply confirms the patient's fears. To be effective, it must neither be a confession which simply makes the patient anxious, nor a denial, which the patient sees as defensive and false. Even when analyst-centred interpretations are successful in creating a sense of containment they leave one with a sense of achievement which is partial and temporary. An impasse may have been evaded, a more friendly relationship with the patient may prevail, but the real work of analysis remains to be done.

The technical challenge is to find an appropriate balance of *patient-centred* and *analyst-centred* interpretations. Interpretations may temporarily have to emphasize containment but ultimately must be concerned with helping the patient gain insight, and an analyst who is perceived as reluctant to pursue this fundamental aim is not experienced as providing containment. Indeed, these two aspects of interpretation can be thought of as feminine and masculine symbols of the analyst's work. Both are required, and insight, which is so often disturbing, is only acceptable to the patient who is held in a containing setting. If the analyst remains sensitive to the patient's reaction to his interpretation and listens to the next piece of material partly as a comment on what has preceded it, then it is possible to shift from one type of interpretation to the other sensitively and flexibly. As development proceeds further, the distinction becomes less important and many interpretations of an intermediate kind become possible, often showing the links between the activity of the patient and the resultant view of the analyst. Such links are impossible to make when the patient is functioning at a more primitive level where containment and being understood take priority over understanding.

Analytic work with borderline and psychotic patients who present such formidable technical problems is always slow and often disheartening but can lead to significant development. Shifts towards the depressive position which are associated with transient emergence from psychic retreats are by no means absent, and if the analyst makes use of these opportunities the patient can use them to gain insight into his use of the retreats and the pathological organizations which underlie them.

References

Abraham, K. (1919) 'A particular form of neurotic resistance against the psychoanalytic method', in *Selected Papers of Karl Abraham*, London: Hogarth Press (1927), 303–11.

—— (1924) 'A short study of the development of the libido, viewed in the light of mental disorders', in *Selected Papers of Karl Abraham*, London: Hogarth Press (1927), 418–501.

Balint, M. (1968) *The Basic Fault: Therapeutic Aspects of Regression*, London: Tavistock.

Berner, P. (1991) 'Delusional atmosphere', *British Journal of Psychiatry*, 159: 88–93.

Bion, W.R. (1957) 'Differentiation of the psychotic from the non-psychotic personalities', *International Journal of Psycho-Analysis*, 38: 266–75; reprinted in *Second Thoughts*, London: Heinemann (1967).

—— (1959) 'Attacks on linking', *International Journal of Psycho-Analysis*, 40: 308–15; reprinted in *Second Thoughts*, London: Heinemann (1967), 93–109.

—— (1962a) *Learning from Experience*, London: Heinemann.

—— (1962b) 'A theory of thinking', *International Journal of Psycho-Analysis*, 43: 306–10; reprinted in *Second Thoughts*, London: Heinemann (1967), 110–19.

—— (1963) *Elements of Psycho-analysis*, London: Heinemann.

—— (1970) *Attention and Interpretation*, London: Tavistock.

Bowlby, J. (1980) *Attachment and Loss*, vol. 3, *Loss, Sadness and Depression*, London: Hogarth Press.

Brenman, E. (1985) 'Cruelty and narrow-mindedness', *International Journal of Psycho-Analysis*, 66: 273–81; reprinted in E. Bott Spillius (1988) *Melanie Klein Today*, vol. 1, *Mainly Theory*, London: Routledge.

Britton, R.S. (1989) 'The missing link: parental sexuality in the Oedipus complex', in *The Oedipus Complex Today*, R.S. Britton, M. Feldman and E. O'Shaughnessy, London: Karnac Books.

—— (1992) 'Keeping things in mind', in *Clinical Lectures on Klein and Bion*, R. Anderson (ed.), London: Routledge.

Britton, R.S., Feldman, M. and O'Shaughnessy, E. (1989) *The Oedipus Complex Today*, London: Karnac Books.

Chasseguet-Smirgel, J. (1974) 'Perversion, idealisation and sublimation', *International Journal of Psycho-Analysis*, 55: 349–57.

—— (1981) 'Loss of reality in perversions – with special reference to fetishism', *Journal of the American Psychoanalytic Association*, 29: 511–34.

—— (1985) *Creativity and Perversion*, London: Free Association Books.

Cooper, A.M. (1986) 'Some limitations on therapeutic effectiveness: the "burnout syndrome"', *The Psychoanalytic Quarterly*, 55: 576–98.

Deutsch, H. (1942) 'Some forms of emotional disturbance and their relationship to schizophrenia', *The Psychoanalytic Quarterly*, 11: 301–21; reprinted in *Neurosis and Character Types*, London: Hogarth Press (1965).

Edmunds, L. and Ingber, R. (1977) 'Psychoanalytical writings on the Oedipus legend: a bibliography', *American Imago*, 34: 374–86.

Fairbairn, R. (1949) 'Steps in the development of an object-relations theory of the personality', *British Journal of Medical Psychology*, 22: 26–31.

Feldman, M. (1989) 'The Oedipus complex: manifestations in the inner world and the therapeutic situation', in *The Oedipus Complex Today*, R.S. Britton, M. Feldman and E. O'Shaughnessy, London: Karnac Books.

—— (1992) 'Splitting and projective identification', in *Clinical Lectures on Klein and Bion*, R. Anderson (ed.), London: Routledge.

Fonagy, P. (1991) 'Thinking about thinking: some clinical and theoretical considerations in the treatment of a borderline patient', *International Journal of Psycho-Analysis*, 72: 639–56.

Fonagy, P. and Moran, G.S. (1991) 'Understanding change in child psychoanalysis', *International Journal of Psycho-Analysis*, 72: 15–22.

Freud, S. (1900) *The Interpretation of Dreams, Standard Edition of the Complete Psychological Works of Sigmund Freud*, SE 4.

—— (1905a) 'Fragment of an analysis of a case of hysteria', SE 7: 3–122.

—— (1905b) *Three Essays on the Theory of Sexuality*, SE 7, 123–243.

—— (1910) 'Leonardo Da Vinci and a memory of his childhood', SE 11: 59–137.

—— (1911a) *Psycho-analytic Notes on an Autobiographic Account of a Case of Paranoia (Dementia Paranoides)*, SE 12: 3–82.

—— (1911b) 'Formulation on the two principles of mental functioning', SE 12: 215–26.

—— (1914) 'On narcissism: an introduction', SE 14: 67–102.

—— (1917) 'Mourning and melancholia', SE 14: 237–58.

—— (1919) '"A child is being beaten", a contribution to the study of sexual perversions', SE 17: 175–204.

—— (1923) *The Ego and the Id*, SE 19: 3–66.

—— (1924) *Neurosis and Psychosis*, SE 19: 149–53.

—— (1927) 'Fetishism', SE 21: 149–57.

—— (1937) 'Analysis terminable and interminable', SE 23: 211–53.

—— (1940) *An Outline of Psycho-analysis*, SE 23: 141–207.

—— (1941) 'Findings, ideas, problems', SE 23: 299–300.

Gillespie, W.H. (1956) 'The general theory of sexual perversion', *International Journal of Psycho-Analysis*, 37: 396–403.

—— (1964) 'The psychoanalytic theory of sexual deviation with special reference to fetishism', in *Sexual Deviation*, I. Rosen (ed.), London: Oxford University Press, 123–45.

Giovacchini, P.L. (1975) *Psychoanalysis of Character Disorders*, New York: Jason Aronson.

—— (1984) *Character Disorders and Adaptive Mechanisms*, New York: Jason Aronson.

Gitelson, M. (1963) 'On the problem of character neurosis', *Journal of the Hillside Hospital*, 12: 3–17.

Glasser, M. (1979) 'Some aspects of the role of aggression in the perversions', in *Sexual Deviation*, I. Rosen (ed.), London: Oxford University Press, 278–305.

—— (1985) '"The weak spot" – some observations on male homosexuality', *International Journal of Psycho-Analysis*, 66: 405–14.

Glover, E. (1933) 'The relation of perversion-formation to the development of reality-sense', *International Journal of Psycho-Analysis*, 14: 486–504; reprinted in E. Glover, *On the Early Development of the Mind*, London: Imago (1956).

—— (1964) 'Aggression and sado-masochism', in *Sexual Deviation*, I. Rosen (ed.), London: Oxford University Press, 146–62.

Green, A. (1987) 'Oedipus, Freud, and us', in *Psychoanalytic Approaches to Literature and Film*, M. Charne and J. Repper (eds), New York: Associated Press, 215–37.

Grosskurth, P. (1986) *Melanie Klein*, London: Hodder & Stoughton.

Grotstein, J.S. (1979) 'The psychoanalytic concept of the borderline organisation', in *Advances in the Psychotherapy of the Borderline Patient*, J. Le Boit and A. Capponi (eds), New York: Jason Aronson.

Guntrip, H. (1968) *Schizoid Phenomena: Object Relations and the Self*, London: Hogarth Press.

Heimann, P. (1950) 'On countertransference', *International Journal of Psycho-Analysis*, 31: 81–4.

—— (1960) 'Countertransference', *British Journal of Medical Psychology*, 33: 9–15.

Jaques, E. (1965) 'Death and the mid-life crisis', *International Journal of Psycho-Analysis*, 46: 502–14.

Joseph, B. (1975) 'The patient who is difficult to reach', in *Tactics and*

Techniques in Psycho-analytic Therapy, vol. II, *Countertransference*, P.L. Giovacchini (ed.), New York: Jason Aronson; reprinted in *Psychic Equilibrium and Psychic Change: Selected Papers of Betty Joseph*, M. Feldman and E. Bott Spillius (eds), London: Routledge (1989).

—— (1981) 'Towards the experiencing of psychic pain', in *'Do I Dare Disturb the Universe? A memorial to W.R. Bion'*, J.S. Grotstein (ed.), Beverly Hills, CA: Caesura Press; reprinted in *Psychic Equilibrium and Psychic Change: Selected Papers of Betty Joseph*, M. Feldman and E. Bott Spillius (eds), London: Routledge (1989).

—— (1982) 'Addiction to near death', *International Journal of Psycho-Analysis*, 63: 449–56; reprinted in *Psychic Equilibrium and Psychic Change: Selected Papers of Betty Joseph*, M. Feldman and E. Bott Spillius (eds), London: Routledge (1989).

—— (1983) 'On understanding and not understanding: some technical issues', *International Journal of Psycho-Analysis*, 64: 291–8; reprinted in *Psychic Equilibrium and Psychic Change: Selected Papers of Betty Joseph*, M. Feldman and E. Bott Spillius (eds), London: Routledge (1989).

—— (1985) 'Transference: the total situation', *International Journal of Psycho-Analysis*, 66: 447–54; reprinted in *Psychic Equilibrium and Psychic Change: Selected Papers of Betty Joseph*, M. Feldman and E. Bott Spillius (eds), London: Routledge (1989).

—— (1989) *Psychic Equilibrium and Psychic Change: Selected Papers of Betty Joseph*, M. Feldman and E. Bott Spillius (eds), London: Routledge.

Kernberg, O.F. (1967) 'Borderline personality organisation', *Journal of the American Psychoanalytic Association*, 15: 641–85.

—— (1975) *Borderline Conditions and Pathological Narcissism*, New York: Jason Aronson.

—— (1976) *Object Relations Theory and Clinical Psychoanalysis*, New York: Jason Aronson.

—— (1979) 'Some implications of object relations theory for psychoanalytic technique', *Journal of the American Psychoanalytic Association*, 27: 207–39.

—— (1983) 'Object relations theory and character analysis', *Journal of the American Psychoanalytic Association*, 31: 247–71.

Khan, M.M.R. (1979) *Alienation in Perversions*, London: Hogarth Press.

Klein, M. (1930) 'The importance of symbol formation in the development of the ego', in *The Writings of Melanie Klein*, vol. 1, London: Hogarth Press (1975), 186–98.

—— (1932) *The Psychoanalysis of Children*, *The Writings of Melanie Klein*, vol. 2, London: Hogarth Press (1975).

—— (1935) 'A contribution to the psychogenesis of manic–depressive states', *International Journal of Psycho-Analysis*, 16: 145–74; reprinted in *The Writings of Melanie Klein*, vol. 1, London: Hogarth Press (1975), 262–89.

—— (1940) 'Mourning and its relation to manic–depressive states', *Inter-*

national Journal of Psycho-Analysis, 21: 125–53; reprinted in *The Writings of Melanie Klein*, vol. 1, London: Hogarth Press (1975), 344–69.

—— (1946) 'Notes on some schizoid mechanisms', *International Journal of Psycho-Analysis*, 27: 99–110; reprinted in *The Writings of Melanie Klein*, vol. 3, London: Hogarth Press (1975), 1–24.

—— (1952) 'Some theoretical conclusions regarding the emotional life of the infant', in *Developments in Psychoanalysis*, J. Riviere (ed.); reprinted in *The Writings of Melanie Klein*, vol. 3, London: Hogarth Press (1975), 61–93.

—— (1955) 'On identification', in *New Directions in Psychoanalysis*, London: Hogarth Press; reprinted in *The Writings of Melanie Klein*, vol. 3, London: Hogarth Press (1975), 141–75.

—— (1957) *Envy and Gratitude*, London: Tavistock; reprinted in *The Writings of Melanie Klein*, vol. 3, London: Hogarth Press (1975), 176–235.

Langs, R. (1978) 'Some communicative properties of the bipersonal field', *International Journal of Psychoanalytic Psychotherapy*, 7: 87–135.

Laufer, M. and Laufer, M.E. (1984) *Adolescence and Developmental Breakdown*, New Haven and London: Yale University Press.

Lax, R.F. (ed.) (1989) *Essential Papers on Character Neurosis and Treatment*, New York: New York University Press.

Lax, R.F., Bach, S. and Burland, J.A. (1980) *Rapprochement: The Critical Subphase of Separation-Individuation*, New York: Jason Aronson.

Leowald, H. (1962) 'Internalisation, separation, mourning, and the super-ego', *The Psychoanalytic Quarterly*, 31: 483–504.

—— (1978) 'Instinct theory, object relations, and psychic-structure formation', *Journal of the American Psychoanalytic Association*, 26: 463–506; reprinted in *Rapprochement: The Critical Subphase of Separation-Individuation*, R.F. Lax, S. Bach and J.A. Burland, New York: Jason Aronson (1980).

Limentani, A. (1976) 'Object choice and actual bisexuality', *International Journal of Psychoanalytic Psychotherapy*, 5: 205–19.

—— (1979) 'The significance of transsexualism in relation to some basic psychoanalytic concepts', *International Review of Psycho-Analysis*, 6: 139–54.

Lindemann, E. (1944) 'Symptomatology and management of acute grief', *American Journal of Psychiatry*, 101: 141–9.

Loewenstein, R.M. (1967) 'Defensive organisation and autonomous ego function', *Journal of the American Psychoanalytic Association*, 15: 795–809.

McDougall, J. (1972) 'Primal scene and sexual perversion', *International Journal of Psycho-Analysis*, 53: 371–84.

Mahler, M., Pine, F. and Bergman, A. (1975) *The Psychological Birth of the Human Infant*, New York: Hutchinson.

Meltzer, D. (1966) 'The relation of anal masturbation to projective identification', *International Journal of Psycho-Analysis*, 47: 335–42.

—— (1968) 'Terror, persecution and dread', *International Journal of Psycho-*

Analysis, 49: 396–401; reprinted in *Sexual States of Mind*, Perthshire: Clunie Press (1973), 99–106.

—— (1973) 'Infantile perverse sexuality', in *Sexual States of Mind*, Perthshire: Clunie Press, 90–8.

Money-Kyrle, R. (1956) 'Normal countertransference and some of its deviations', *International Journal of Psycho-Analysis*, 37: 360–6; reprinted in *The Collected Papers of Roger Money-Kyrle*, Perthshire: Clunie Press (1978), 330–42.

—— (1968) 'Cognitive development', *International Journal of Psycho-Analysis*, 49: 691–8; reprinted in *The Collected Papers of Roger Money-Kyrle*, Perthshire: Clunie Press (1978), 416–33.

—— (1971) 'The aim of psycho-analysis', *International Journal of Psycho-Analysis*, 52: 103–6; reprinted in *The Collected Papers of Roger Money-Kyrle*, Perthshire: Clunie Press (1978), 442–9.

Nunberg, H.G. (1956) 'Character and neurosis', *International Journal of Psycho-Analysis*, 37: 36–45.

O'Shaughnessy, E. (1981) 'A clinical study of a defensive organisation', *International Journal of Psycho-Analysis*, 62: 359–69.

—— (1993) 'Enclaves and excursions', *International Journal of Psycho-Analysis*, 73: 603–11.

Parkes, C.M. (1972) *Bereavement: Studies of Grief in Adult Life*, London: Tavistock.

Pilikian, H.I. (1974) Interview with Douglas Keay, following production of *Oedipus Rex* in Chichester, *Guardian*, 17 July.

Potamianou, A. (1992) *Un Bouclier dans l'economie des etats – limites: l'espoir*, Paris: Presses Universitaires de France.

Racker, H. (1957) 'The meaning and uses of countertransference', *The Psychoanalytic Quarterly*, 26: 303–57; reprinted in *Transference and Countertransference*, London: Hogarth Press (1968).

Reich, W. (1933) *Character Analysis*, New York: Orgone Institute Press (1949).

Rey, J.H. (1975) 'Liberté et processus de pensée psychotique', *La Vie Médicale au Canada Français*, 4: 1046–60.

—— (1979) 'Schizoid phenomena in the borderline', in *Advances in the Psychotherapy of the Borderline Patient*, J. Le Boit and A. Capponi (eds), New York: Jason Aronson.

—— (1986) 'Reparation', *Journal of the Melanie Klein Society*, 4: 5–35.

—— (1988) 'That which patients bring to analysis', *International Journal of Psycho-Analysis*, 69: 457–70.

Riesenberg-Malcolm, R. (1981) 'Expiation as a defence', *International Journal of Psychoanalytic Psychotherapy*, 8: 549–70.

Riviere, J. (1936) 'A contribution to the analysis of the negative therapeutic reaction', *International Journal of Psycho-Analysis*, 17: 304–20; reprinted in A. Hughes (ed.), *The Inner World and Joan Riviere: Collected Papers 1920–1958*, London: Karnac (1991), 134–53.

Rosenfeld, H.A. (1950) 'Notes on the psychopathology of confusional states in chronic schizophrenia', *International Journal of Psycho-Analysis*, 31: reprinted in *Psychotic States*, London: Hogarth Press (1965).

—— (1964) 'On the psychopathology of narcissism: a clinical approach', *International Journal of Psycho-Analysis*, 45: 332–7; reprinted in *Psychotic States*, London: Hogarth Press (1965).

—— (1971a) 'A clinical approach to the psychoanalytic theory of the life and death instincts: an investigation into the aggressive aspects of narcissism', *International Journal of Psycho-Analysis*, 52: 169–78.

—— (1971b) 'Contributions to the psychopathology of psychotic patients: the importance of projective identification in the ego structure and object relations of the psychotic patient', in *Problems of Psychosis*, P. Doucet and C. Laurin (eds), Amsterdam: Excerpta Medica; reprinted in E. Bott Spillius (1988), *Melanie Klein Today*, vol. 1, *Mainly Theory*, London: Routledge.

—— (1978) 'Some therapeutic factors in psycho-analysis', *International Journal of Psycho-analysis and Psycho-therapy*, 7: 152–64.

—— (1983) 'Primitive object relations', *International Journal of Psycho-Analysis*, 64: 261–7.

—— (1987) *Impasse and Interpretation*, London: Tavistock.

Rudnytsky, P.L. (1987) *Freud and Oedipus*, New York: Columbia University Press.

Sachs, H. (1923) 'On the genesis of perversions', *Internationale Zeitschrift für Psycho-Analyse*, 19: 172–82; republished in C.W. Socarides, *Homosexuality*, New York: Jason Aronson (1978); translated by Hella Freud Bernays.

Sandler, J. (1976) 'Countertransference and role-responsiveness', *International Review of Psycho-Analysis*, 3: 43–7.

Sandler, J. and Sandler, A.M. (1978) 'On the development of object relationships and affects', *International Journal of Psycho-Analysis*, 59: 285–96.

Segal, H. (1956) 'Depression in the schizophrenic', *International Journal of Psycho-Analysis*, 37: 339–43; reprinted in *The Work of Hanna Segal*, New York: Jason Aronson (1981), 121–30.

—— (1957) 'Notes on symbol formation', *International Journal of Psycho-Analysis*, 38: 391–7; reprinted in *The Work of Hanna Segal*, New York: Jason Aronson (1981), 49–65.

—— (1958) 'Fear of death: notes on the analysis of an old man', *International Journal of Psycho-Analysis*, 39: 187–91; reprinted in *The Work of Hanna Segal*, New York: Jason Aronson (1981), 173–82.

—— (1964) *Introduction to the Work of Melanie Klein*, London: Hogarth Press.

—— (1972) 'A delusional system as a defence against the re-emergence of a catastrophic situation', *International Journal of Psycho-Analysis*, 53: 393–401.

—— (1983) 'Some clinical implications of Melanie Klein's work: emergence from narcissism', *International Journal of Psycho-Analysis*, 64: 269–76.

—— (1991) *Dream, Phantasy, and Art*, London: Routledge.

Shengold, L. (1988) *Halo in the Sky*, New York: Guildford Press.
—— (1989) *Soul Murder: The Effects of Childhood Abuse and Deprivation*, New Haven, CT: Yale University Press.
Shorter Oxford English Dictionary (1933) London: Oxford University Press.
Sims, A. (1988) *Symptoms in the Mind: An Introduction to Descriptive Psychopathology*, London: Baillière Tindall.
Socarides, C.W. (1978) *Homosexuality*, New York: Jason Aronson.
Sohn, L. (1985) 'Narcissistic organisation, projective identification and the formation of the identificate', *International Journal of Psycho-Analysis*, 66: 201–14; reprinted in E. Bott Spillius (1988) *Melanie Klein Today*, vol. 1, *Mainly Theory*, London: Routledge.
Spillius, E. Bott (1983) 'Some developments from the work of Melanie Klein', *International Journal of Psycho-Analysis*, 64: 321–32.
—— (1988a) *Melanie Klein Today*, vol. 1, *Mainly Theory*, London: Routledge.
—— (1988b) *Melanie Klein Today*, vol. 2, *Mainly Practice*, London: Routledge.
Steiner, J. (1979) 'The border between the paranoid-schizoid and the depressive positions in the borderline patient', *British Journal of Medical Psychology*, 52: 385–91.
—— (1982) 'Perverse relationships between parts of the self: a clinical illustration', *International Journal of Psycho-Analysis*, 63: 241–51.
—— (1985) 'Turning a blind eye: the cover-up for Oedipus', *International Review of Psycho-Analysis*, 12: 161–72.
—— (1987) 'The interplay between pathological organisations and the paranoid-schizoid and depressive positions', *International Journal of Psycho-Analysis*; reprinted in E. Bott Spillius (1988) *Melanie Klein Today*, vol. 1, *Mainly Theory*, London: Routledge.
—— (1989a) 'The aim of psychoanalysis', *Psychoanalytic Psychotherapy*, 4: 109–20.
—— (1989b) 'The psychoanalytic contribution of Herbert Rosenfeld', *International Journal of Psycho-Analysis*, 70: 611–17.
—— (1990a) 'Pathological organisations as obstacles to mourning: the role of unbearable guilt', *International Journal of Psycho-Analysis*, 71: 87–94.
—— (1990b) 'The retreat from truth to omnipotence in *Oedipus at Colonus*', *International Review of Psycho-Analysis*, 17: 227–37.
—— (1990c) 'The defensive function of pathological organisations', in *Master Clinicians on Treating the Regressed Patient*, B.L. Boyer and P. Giovacchini (eds), New York: Jason Aronson.
—— (1991) 'A psychotic organisation of the personality', *International Journal of Psycho-Analysis*, 72: 201–7.
—— (1992) 'The equilibrium between the paranoid-schizoid and the depressive positions', in *Clinical Lectures on Klein and Bion*, Robin Anderson (ed.), London: Routledge.

Stewart, H. (1961) 'Jocasta's crimes', *International Journal of Psycho-Analysis*, 42: 424–30.

Stoller, R. (1975) *Perversion: The Erotic Form of Hatred*, Brighton: Harvester Press.

Vellacott, P. (1956) *Aeschylus: The Oresteian Trilogy*, Harmondsworth: Penguin Books.

—— (1961) *Aeschylus: Prometheus Bound and Other Plays*, Harmondsworth: Penguin Books.

—— (1971) *Sophocles and Oedipus: A Study of* Oedipus Tyrannus *with a New Translation*, London: Macmillan.

—— (1978) '*Oedipus at Colonus:* An alternate view', Unpublished manuscript.

Watling, E.F. (1947) *The Theban Plays*, Harmondsworth: Penguin Books.

Winnicott, D.W. (1953) 'Transitional objects and transitional phenomena: a study of the first not-me possession', *International Journal of Psycho-Analysis*, 34: 89–97.

—— (1958) *Collected Papers: Through Paediatrics to Psycho-Analysis*, London: Tavistock.

—— (1960) 'Ego distortions in terms of true and false self', in *The Maturational Process and the Facilitating Environment*, London: Hogarth Press (1965), 140–57.

—— (1965) *The Maturational Process and the Facilitating Environment*, London: Hogarth Press.

—— (1969) 'The use of an object', *International Journal of Psycho-Analysis*, 50: 711–16; reprinted in *Playing and Reality* (1971), London: Tavistock.

—— (1971) *Playing and Reality*, London: Tavistock.

Winnington-Ingram, R.P. (1980) *Sophocles: An Interpretation*, Cambridge: Cambridge University Press.

Name index

Abraham, K. 4, 40, 43, 47

Balint, M. 41
Berner, P. 66
Bion, W.R. 95; on attacks on
  perceptual apparatus 64; bizarre
  objects 30, 6; containment 8,
  59–60, 140; equilibrium P/S ↔
  D 28; evasion or modification of
  anxiety 67; parts of the personality
  5, 67–9; pathological
  fragmentation 29; projective
  identification, violence of 7;
  restitution of ego 66; return of
  projections 60; reversible
  projective identification 67
Bowlby, J. 60
Brenman, E. 46
Britton, R.S. 89, 97; on containment
  42; need for third object 140

Chasseguet-Smirgel, J. 89, 98
Cooper, A.M. 41

Deutsch, H. 41

Edmunds, L. on bibliography of
  Oedipus myth 117

Fairbairn, R. 52
Feldman, M. 89
Fonagy, P. 42, 68
Freud, S. on artful reconciliation of

contradiction 93; bereavement 59;
co-existence of psychotic and
non-psychotic 67; death instinct 4,
40, 45; Dora case 17; fetishism 12,
88–94, 99; having and being the
object 34; Leonardo case 6, 42–3;
mourning 34–5; mourning and
detachment of libido 61; narcissism
40–3; patch over rent in ego 65;
perversion 90; perversion as the
negative of neurosis 100; rent in
the ego in psychosis 64; Schreber
case 49, 65; two parts of the
personality 67

Gillespie, W.H. 90
Giovacchini, P.L. 41
Gitelson, M. 41
Glasser, M. 90
Glover, E. 99
Green, A. 120
Grosskurth, P. 36
Grotstein, J.S. 104
Guntrip, H. 52

Heimann, P. on counter-transference
  140

Ingber, R. on bibliography of
  Oedipus myth 117

Jaques, E. 129
Joseph, B. on defensive systems 4;

156

Subject index

actualization 140
anal world 98
analyst: at cross purposes with patient 131; capacity to think 62; drawn into the organization 104; independence of 62; under pressure 3; undermining confidence and integrity of 81
analyst-centred interpretations 131–44; difficulties of 145
Antigone and goodness 128
Apollo 120, 121, 125
artful reconciliation of contradiction 92

balanced introjection and projection 67
bereavement and mourning 60
betrayal: as a cause of indignation 82
bizarre objects 30, 65
borderline: mental structure 52; patients 1, 3, 5, 41, 52–3; 143; position 2, 11; traumatized patient 42

catastrophic situation, defences against 48
character armour 4, 40, 43
character disorder and resistance 41
claustro-agoraphobic dilemma 53
clinical material: Mrs A 14–21, 100; Mrs B 55–9; Mr C 69–72, 102–34; Mr D 77–80, 101; Mr E 80–2, 101–2; Mr F 105–14; Mrs G 135–9; Patient A 31; Patient B 32; Patient C 36–8; Patient D 38–9
collusion: and cover-up 129
combined object 97
confrontation: with the organization 9; with reality 128
confusion: between good and bad 97; and panic 30, 49, 50, 105; between self and object 27; between the sexes 97; defences against 30, 32, 57, 65, 113–14
confusional states: and breakdown of splitting 112; and envy 30
containment: and being understood 141; dependence on presence of the object 60; failure of 132, 141, 145; giving rise to integration 60; necessary but not sufficient for development 141, 143; by the organization 7, 9; priority over understanding 146; problems of 61; and projective identification 42, 132, 140
contempt for truth 129
counter-transference 132; difficulties with 140; unreliability of 140
co-existence of contradictions 91
Creon 118–21
cruelty and tyranny 44

deadness: fascination with 16
death instinct: and destructive narcissism 45; Klein's views on 26; and obstacles to analysis 40; and

159